AF250998

Neonatal Medicine

Edited by Antonina I. Chubarova

Published in London, United Kingdom

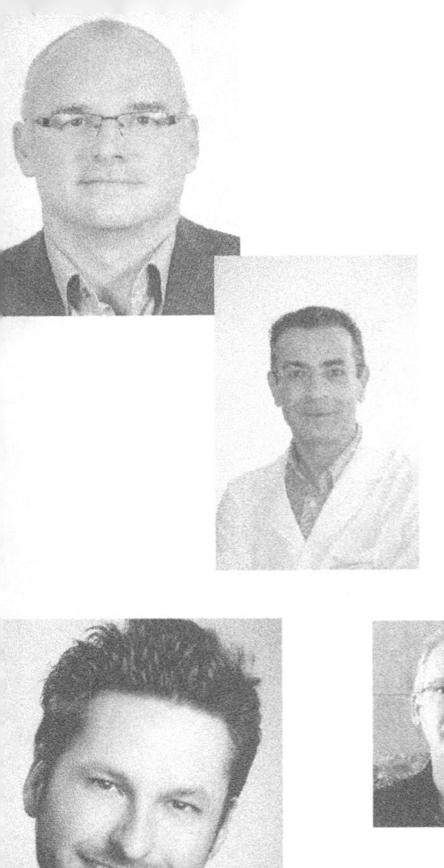
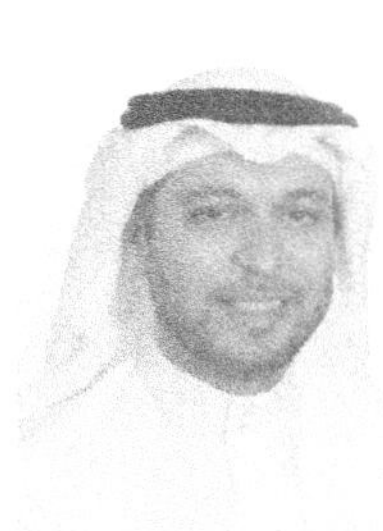
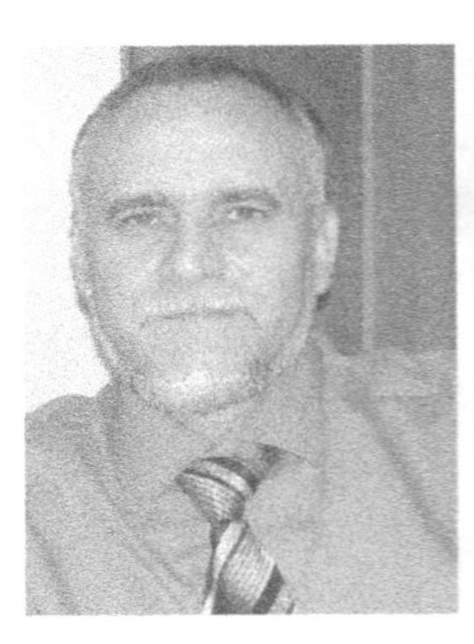
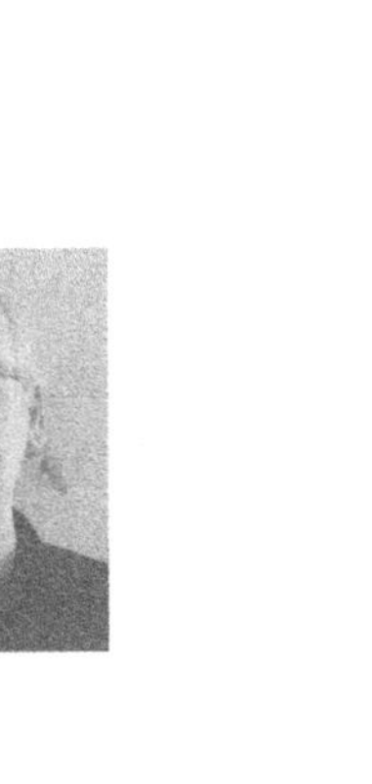
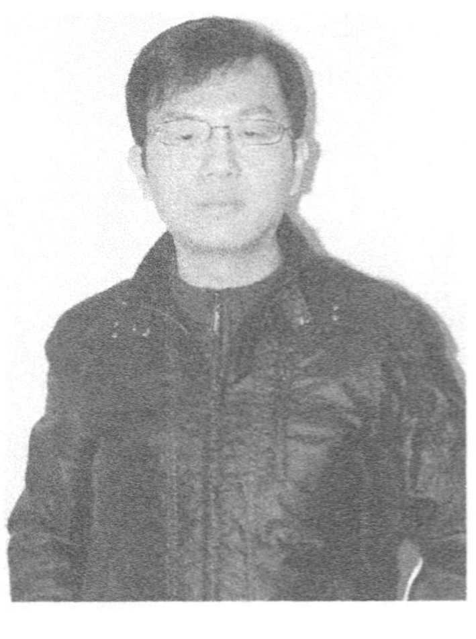
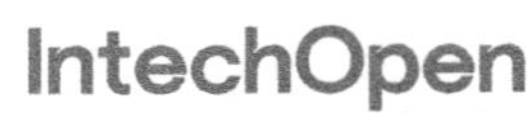

IntechOpen

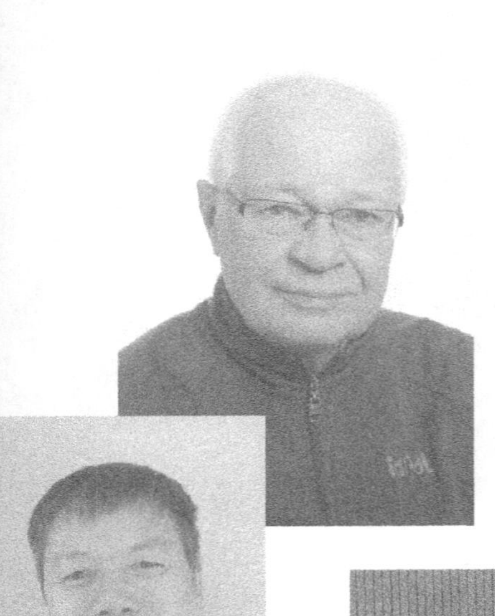
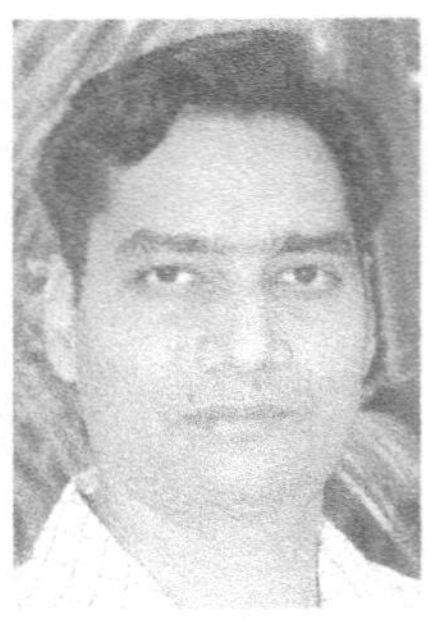
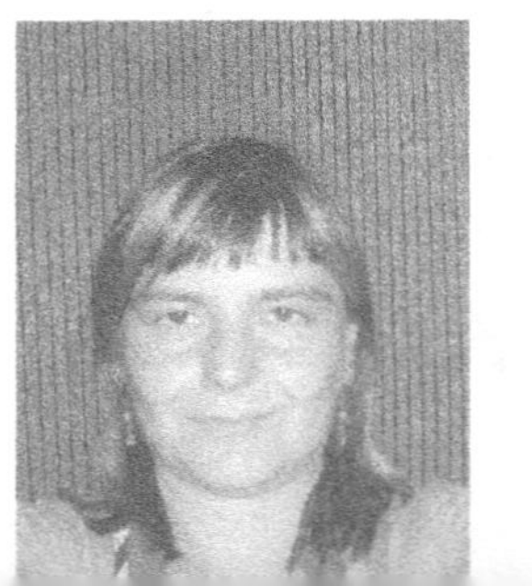
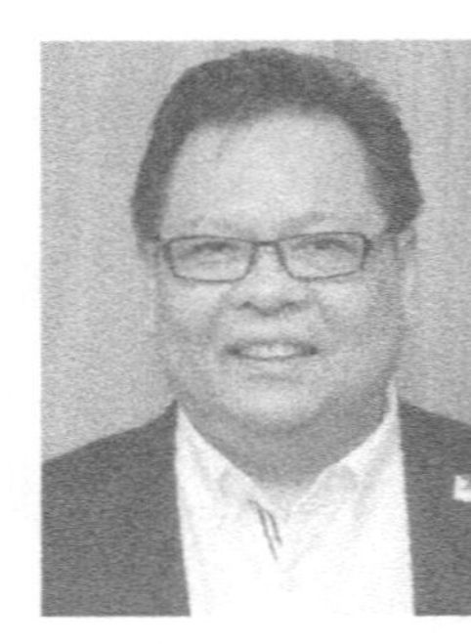
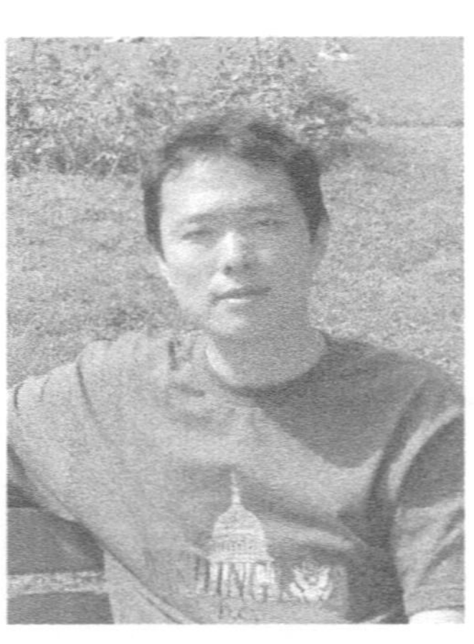

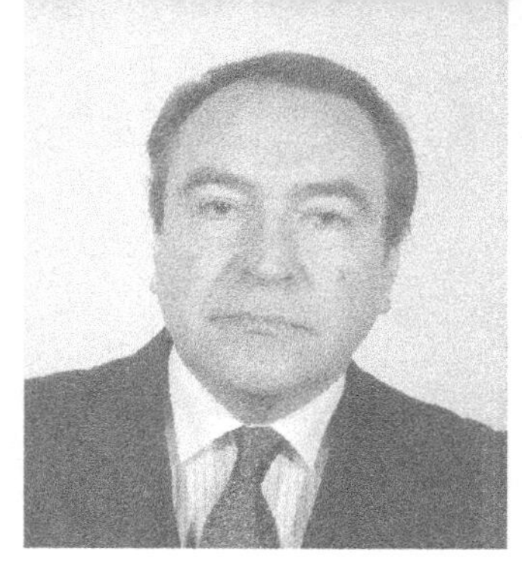
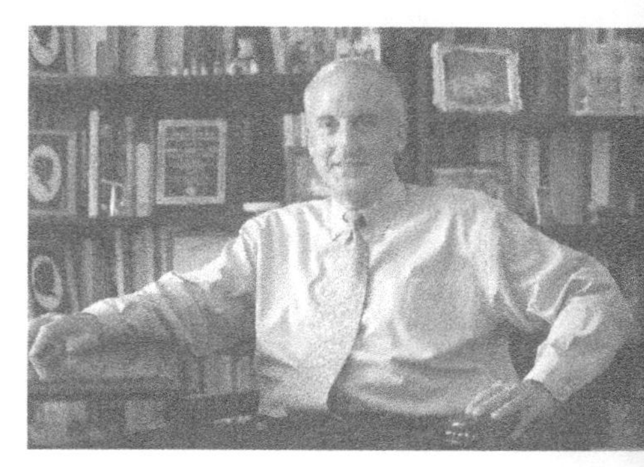
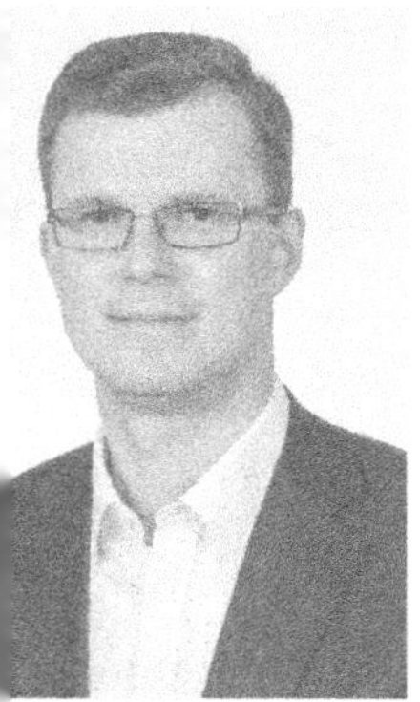
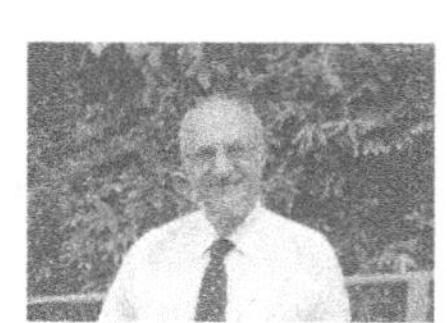
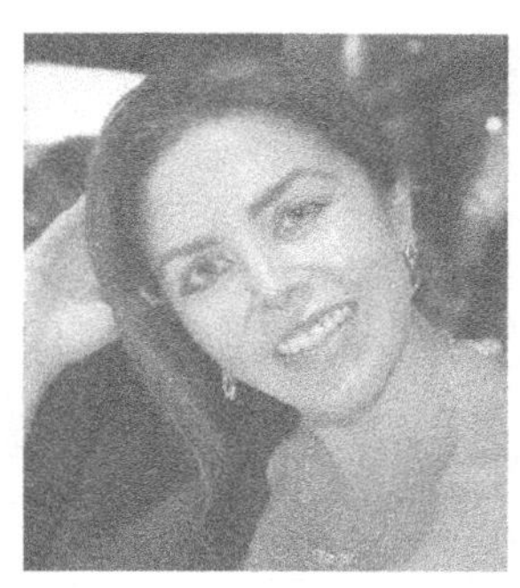

Supporting open minds since 2005

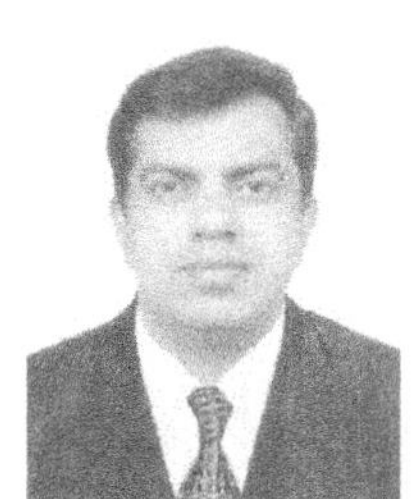
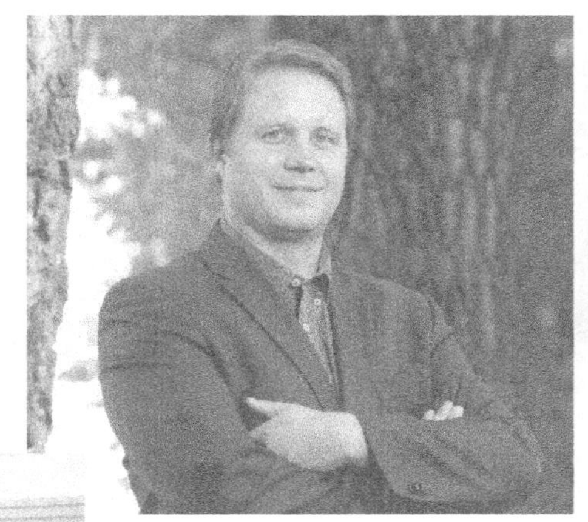
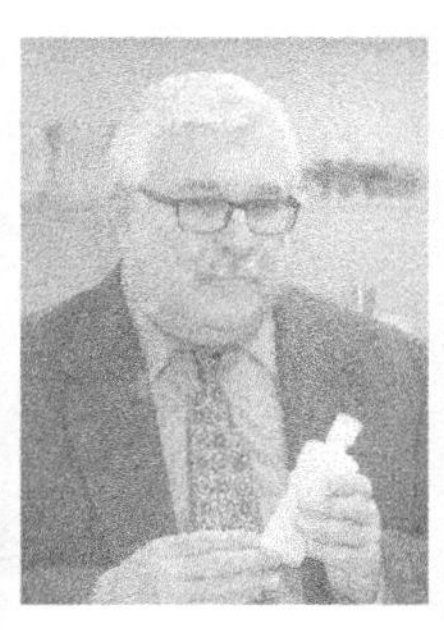
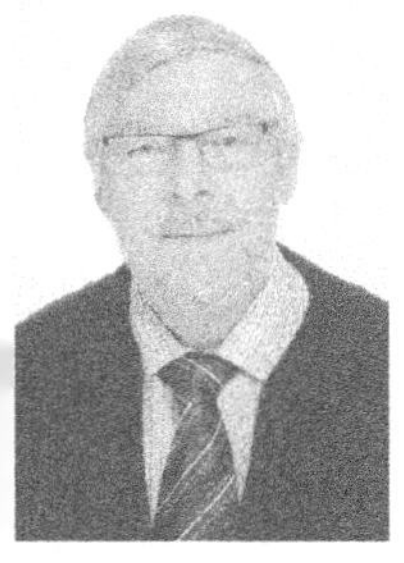
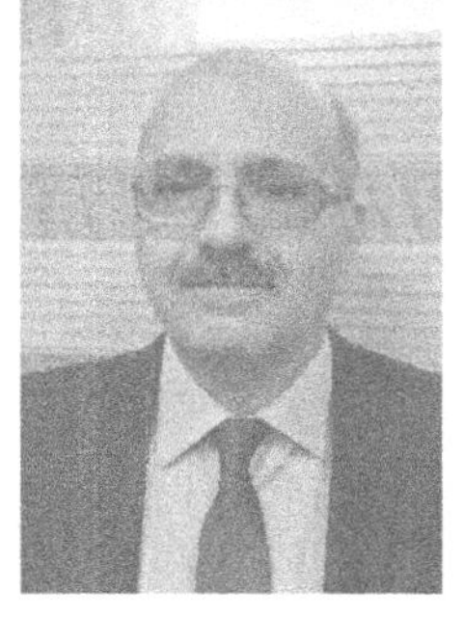
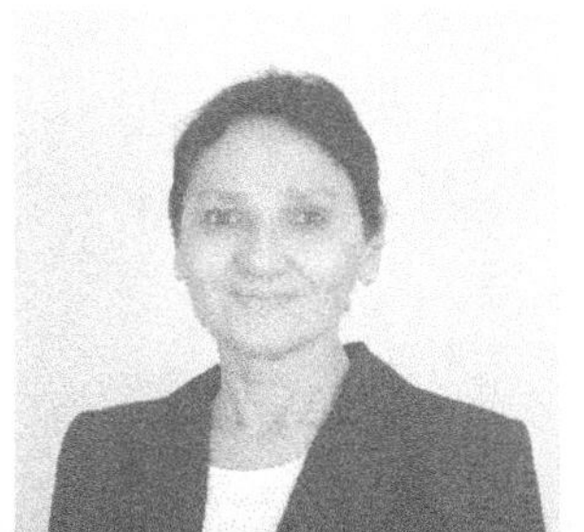
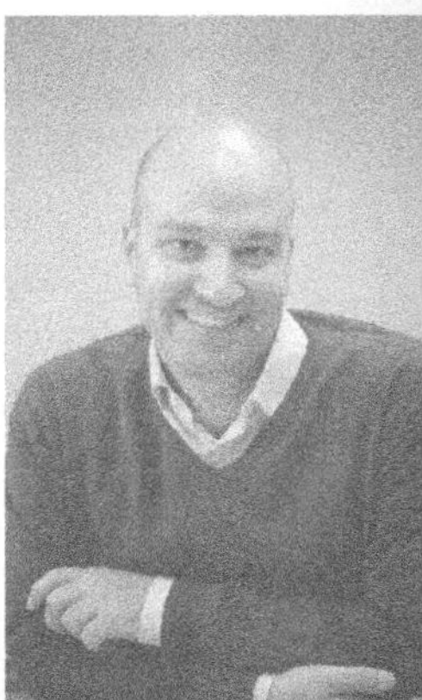

Neonatal Medicine
http://dx.doi.org/10.5772/intechopen.76552
Edited by Antonina I. Chubarova

Contributors
Simona Delia Nicoara, J. Wells Logan, Omid Fathi, Roopali Bapat, Edward Shepherd, Thillagavathie Pillay, Danilo Boskovic, Ijeoma Esiaba, Danilyn Angeles, Mehmet Şah İpek, Antonina I. Chubarova

Notice
Statements and opinions expressed in the chapters are these of the individual contributors and not necessarily those of the editors or publisher. No responsibility is accepted for the accuracy of information contained in the published chapters. The publisher assumes no responsibility for any damage or injury to persons or property arising out of the use of any materials, instructions, methods or ideas contained in the book.

First published in London, United Kingdom, 2019 by IntechOpen
IntechOpen is the global imprint of INTECHOPEN LIMITED, registered in England and Wales, registration number: 11086078, The Shard, 25th floor, 32 London Bridge Street
London, SE19SG – United Kingdom
Printed in Croatia

British Library Cataloguing-in-Publication Data
A catalogue record for this book is available from the British Library

Additional hard and PDF copies can be obtained from orders@intechopen.com

Neonatal Medicine
Edited by Antonina I. Chubarova
p. cm.
Print ISBN 978-1-83962-274-8
Online ISBN 978-1-83962-275-5
eBook (PDF) ISBN 978-1-83962-276-2

Meet the editor

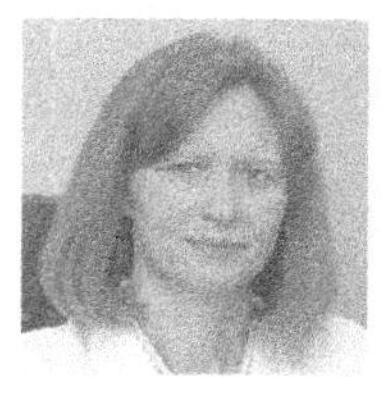

Dr. Antonina I. Chubarova is Medical Director of the Children's City Clinical Hospital N13 named after Filatov N.F., Moscow, Russia, and Chair Professor of the Paediatrics Hospital named after Tabolin V.A. of the Russian National Research Medical University named after Pirogov N.I. Her education and previous work posts and accomplishments include: 1985–1991 pediatric faculty of the 2nd Moscow Medical Institute; 1991 MD in pediatrics; 1991–1993 clinical resident in pediatrics; 1996 PhD in Medicine (thesis: Morphology and function of small intestine mucosa in infants with central nervous system disorders); 1997–1999 pediatrician at City Hospital N 67, Moscow; professor's assistant Chair of Child Diseases of the Russian State Medical University; 2000–2007 associate professor; 2007 thesis: Clinical and pathogenic basis of nutritional support in perinatology; and 2012–2015 Vice Medical Director of the Children's City Hospital named after Bashlyaeva Z.A.

Contents

Preface

Maternal and neonatal care technologies have been developing quickly over the last few decades.

The reason for this activity is the vast influence of neonatal care on the future economic stability of society; no other specialties of medicine have that influence on human resources. It is not now just a question of saving lives. It is a question of the possibilities of programming the future quality of life, somatic and mental disease rates, socialization, and life expectancy. New possibilities of respiratory support, instrumental and laboratory monitoring, and new materials are playing a big role in decreasing neonatal and infant mortality. The earliest period of infant life is called the "golden hours" because the sophisticated application of new technologies can save life and reduce negative consequences for the future.

Another trend associated with technological evolution is the humanization of care. Creating a friendly atmosphere in hospitals, parent involvement in neonatal care, and reducing mothers' anxieties are simple but effective methods for improving child health.

The external factors that are interacting with an organism can play a role in programming stimulus if they act in that special critical period of differentiation of tissues and the forming of functions. For humans the perinatal and neonatal periods are the most important in epigenetic programming. Epigenetic mechanisms can regulate gene activity and create stability for all future life. The most important epigenetic mechanisms are methylation, histone modification, and miRNA and tiRNA pathways.

By means of simple environmental factors like nutrition, oxygen support, mothers' behavior, and others metabolic and immune pathways can be programmed for the future. We now understand why throughout life the most important period is infancy, especially the neonatal period.

This book combines different aspects of perinatal care that can be of enormous importance for the health of future generations.

Antonina Chubarova
Professor
Pirogov Russian National Research Medical University,
Russia

Introductory Chapter: Neonatology - Combining Intensive Care and Family-Friendly Atmosphere

Antonina Chubarova

1. Introduction

The new millennium is of course the epoch of technologies. New technologies are already everywhere in our life: information technologies, reproductive technologies, new materials, and world globalization. What can this lead to in the inner world of mother and child, in everlasting mystery of childbirth, and in the struggle of physicians for every lifesaving?

This book combines different chapters united by the same idea to improve medical aid to neonate and its parents by the means of modern technologies.

Each of them gives an overview of a very important area of perinatology beginning from technologies applied during the first minutes of life till methods that help family to be socialized.

It is very important to know that perinatal period is a period of adaptation of fetus and child organism to the environment. "Adaptation" means changes in genes working that will allow a child to have the most advantageous metabolism and behavior in future life. The more we know about genotype, the more it is clear that it is not the only one factor that determines phenotype. The environmental factors such as nutrition, microbiota, mother's behavior, and others can be the strong regulators of gene work. Such factors are called epigenetic factors. During some periods of intensive changes of gene activity, the so-called critical window, these factors can lead to permanent changes in gene activity and form a phenotype. In other words epigenetic factors have a programming role in critical periods. The patterns of reaction to infection, stress, food deprivation, and other environmental factors in later periods of life including aging are formed in gestational period and neonatal period. Perinatal period is the most important critical period in mammal's life. It is a period when the health of future generations can be programmed for all the life period [1].

The mechanisms of programming are already discovered. The process of gene methylation is called "the prima donna" of epigenetic. Methylation inactivates gene transcription [2]. In embryo before implantation, the majority of genes are methylated, and all the next development is a series of demethylation and methylation. Other mechanisms are histone modifications, regulatory miRNA, and tiRNA [3, 4].

Nutrition is a strong external factor of programming. It is a signal of availability of nutrient resources, their quantity and quality [5]. Nutrition contains methyl ($-CH_3$) group donors: folates, B12, B6, choline, methionine, and betaine. Also nutrition is a platform for macro- and microorganism interaction. And finally it is a functional molecular donor and direct regulator of gene function.

The mother's under- and overnutrition can lead to placenta regulatory gene changes. The placenta can, for example, increase glucose transport to fetus, but in some critical situations, its functioning may be "selfish" through accumulating nutrients for its own needs [6]. The placenta regulates also the synthesis of neuroactive factors, serving as a major source of serotonin to the fetal forebrain [7].

In the fetus itself, major changes following nutrition impairment are happening in genes and their products regulating reaction to stress, fat, and glucose metabolism [8, 9]. Is now shown in big cohort studies that body composition, rate of metabolic syndrome, obesity, atherosclerosis, type 2 diabetes, and rate of cardiovascular death depend on nutrition in prenatal period and infancy [10]. For example in the population of the survivors of Dutch Hunger Winter at the age of 60–65, birth weight negatively correlated with the rate of glucose intolerance, hyperlipidemia, and arterial hypertension, and there was found less DNA methylation of the maternally imprinted IGF2 gene [11, 12]. Learning ability, behavior, and fertility in adult life are also dependent on nutrition in critical period [13–15]. Psychiatric diseases are also partially programmed by continuous dietary deficiency by inactivation of expression of genes for myelin development and oligodendrocyte-related genes [16].

What can we do to regulate undesirable effects of complicated pregnancy? We should know that the infancy period is also a critical period and neonatologists and other specialists can do a lot to regulate future development, especially in premature neonates.

It is important to minimize stressful factors such as hypo- and hyperoxia, pain, and caloric and protein deficit. The moment of adaptation to extrauterine life is of a great importance. The first hours of life are "golden hours," and they are important not only in the context of lifesaving but in the context of programming.

After birth nutritional programming continues through nutrients, regulatory factors, and microflora of milk, but there are specific ways of continuing direct gene regulation through microvesicles containing mRNA transcripts, which possess reverse transcriptase activity [17].

To provide breast milk feeding [18] with or without combination with artificial parenteral or enteral nutrition, to take care of forming microbiota [19], is a way to prevent a big number of negative metabolic changes.

Finally, the mothers' behavior and her integration in child care also have a programming effect. Animal experiments and big cohort studies [20–22] showed that less anxious and more positive mother more often takes a child and contacts with him or her and this has enormous effect on offspring's reaction to stress in cognitive development in future life.

This book gives an overview of modern strategies in neonatology that can influence health of adult.

Author details

Antonina Chubarova
Pirogov Russian National Research Medical University, Russia

*Address all correspondence to: ach-12@yandex.ru

IntechOpen

References

[1] Waterland RA. Epigenetic mechanisms and gastrointestinal development. The Journal of Pediatrics. 2006;**149**(5 Suppl):S137-S142

[2] Santos KF, Mazzola TN, Carvalho HF. The prima donna of epigenetics: The regulation of gene expression by DNA methylation. Brazilian Journal of Medical and Biological Research. 2005;**38**(10):1531-1541

[3] Junien C, Gallou-Kabani C, Vigé A, Gross MS. Nutritional epigenomics: Consequences of unbalanced diets on epigenetics processes of programming during lifespan and between generations. Annales d'endocrinologie. 2005;**66**(2 Pt 3):2S19-2S28

[4] Holliday R. Epigenetics: A historical overview. Epigenetics. 2006;**1**(2):76-80

[5] Mathers JC. Early Nutrition: Impact on Epigenetics. Forum of Nutrition. 2007;**60**:42-48

[6] Hsiao EY, Patterson PH. Placental regulation of maternal-fetal interactions and brain development. Developmental Neurobiology. 2012;**72**(10):1317-1326

[7] Fowden AL. The placenta and intrauterine programming. Journal of Neuroendocrinology. 2008;**20**:439-450

[8] Burdge GC, Hanson MA, Slater-Jefferies JL, Lillycrop KA. Epigenetic regulation of transcription: A mechanism for inducing variations in phenotype (fetal programming) by differences in nutrition during early life? The British Journal of Nutrition. 2007;**97**(6):1036-1046

[9] Myatt L. Placental adaptive responses and fetal programming. The Journal of Physiology. 2006;**572**(Pt 1):25-30

[10] Langley-Evans SC. Developmental programming of health and disease. The Proceedings of the Nutrition Society. 2006;**65**(1):97-105

[11] Stanner SA, Yudkin JS. Fetal programming and the Leningrad Siege study. Twin Research. 2001;**4**:287-292

[12] Roseboom TJ, van der Meulen JH, Ravelli AC, Osmond C, Barker DJ, Bleker OP. Effects of prenatal exposure to the Dutch famine on adult disease in later life: An overview. Twin Research. 2001;**4**:293-298

[13] Walker CD. Nutritional aspects modulating brain development and the responses to stress in early neonatal life. Progress in Neuro-Psychopharmacology & Biological Psychiatry. 2005;**29**(8):1249-1263

[14] Saugstad LF. From superior adaptation and function to brain dysfunction—The neglect of epigenetic factors. Nutrition and Health. 2004;**18**(1):3-27

[15] Ramakrishnan U, Grant F, Goldenberg T, Zongrone A, Martorell R. Effect of women's nutrition before and during early pregnancy on maternal and infant outcomes: A systematic review. Paediatric and Perinatal Epidemiology. 2012;**26**(s1):285-301

[16] Casper RC. Nutrients, neurodevelopment, and mood. Current Psychiatry Reports. 2004;**6**(6):425-429

[17] Irmak MK. Integration of maternal genome into the neonate genome through breast milk mRNA transcripts and reverse transcriptase. Theoretical Biology & Medical Modelling. 2012;**9**:20

[18] Fernandez-Twinn DS, Ozanne SE. Early life nutrition and metabolic programming. Annals of the New York Academy of Sciences. 2010;**1212**:78-96

[19] Grenham S, Clarke G, Cryan JF, Dinan TG. Brain–gut–microbe

communication in health and disease.
Frontiers in Physiology. 2011;**2**:94

[20] Mulder C, Kain J, Uauy R, Seidell JC.
Maternal attitudes and child-feeding
practices: Relationship with the BMI
of Chilean children. Nutrition Journal.
2009;**8**:37

[21] Viltart O, Vanbesien-Mailliot CC.
Impact of prenatal stress on
neuroendocrine programming.
ScientificWorldJournal.
2007;**7**:1493-1537

[22] Quah PL, Fries LR, Chan MJ.
Validation of the children's eating
behavior questionnaire in 5 and 6 year-
old children: The GUSTO Cohort Study.
Frontiers in Psychology. 2019;**10**:824

Chapter 2

Golden Hours: An Approach to Postnatal Stabilization and Improving Outcomes

Omid Fathi, Roopali Bapat, Edward G. Shepherd and John Wells Logan

Abstract

The "Golden Hour" model of care originated in adult trauma medicine. Recently, this concept has been applied to premature neonates and the care they receive immediately after birth. This is not limited to the first hour of life, however, as this approach encompasses the first hours and days after birth. While no universal description defines the Golden Hour model, critical domains include initial delivery room management, thermoregulation, ventilation and oxygenation, glycemic control and prevention of infection. Strong evidence favors standardization of care to improve short- and long-term outcomes. This approach to care for the most at-risk premature infant is typically institution-specific; thus, team-building and quality improvement are critical to the care of these vulnerable patients.

Keywords: Golden Hour, prematurity, preterm, neonate, extremely low birth weight infant, resuscitation, quality improvement

1. History and introduction

The "Golden Hour" concept derives from the adult trauma literature, and generally describes the period after a traumatic injury during which prompt medical attention is needed to prevent death. The term was first introduced by a military surgeon, R. Adams Cowley. Cowley's research was directed primarily at the management of post-traumatic shock. According to Cowley, shock is a "momentary pause" in the pathway leading to death, and the "golden hour" is that period in which life-saving interventions can be initiated to prevent death or extreme morbidity. Cowley's research was instrumental in the study of shock and trauma in the United States, and his contribution has influenced the care of high-risk newborns as well.

For over a decade, neonatologists have been applying this concept to the care of high-risk newborns in the neonatal intensive care unit (NICU) [1]. However, the Golden Hour conveys a slightly different meaning in the NICU. In the NICU, the term generally refers to the first few hours immediately after birth. High-quality, timely, and efficient care, initiated within the Golden Hour window, can mitigate at least some of the risks associated with high-risk newborn care. Golden Hour protocols generally include standards and guidelines based on available evidence that can decrease morbidity and mortality. Here we discuss the Golden Hour concept for care of preterm infants, especially those born less than 28 weeks post-menstrual age

(PMA). Extremely preterm newborns are highly vulnerable to complications in the early postnatal period, and adherence to best-evidence standards or guidelines can improve both survival and neurodevelopmental outcomes [2].

The aim of a Golden Hour protocol in the NICU is to apply evidence to clinical practice as safely and efficiently as possible. While the term "Golden Hour" implies the first 60 minutes after birth, the first several hours to days are critical as well [3]. The care of each infant must be individualized, but the Golden Hour concept emphasizes preparedness and adherence to guidelines with the aim of improving the quality of care. One author described the Golden Hour as a "philosophical approach" that reinforces communications, evidence-based protocols and procedures, and standardizes as many elements as possible with the aim of improving care and outcomes [2].

The outcomes improved by Golden Hour care are those most important to parents: survival, chronic lung disease, hearing and vision, and long-term neurodevelopment [3]. Early postnatal metrics are essential in the development of Golden Hour protocols, and there is strong evidence that improving specific components of care improves long-term outcomes as well. Among the most important of these are delivery-room practices such as teamwork, leadership, and communication, the use of oxygen and positive pressure ventilation, hemodynamic management, maintenance of a thermo-neutral environment, glycemic control, and identification and management of infectious risk factors.

While there are no randomized controlled trials evaluating any one comprehensive Golden Hour protocol, there is ample support for the use of evidence-based standards in several clinical domains unique to the early postnatal period. One report of a standardized protocol demonstrated a 67% reduction in mortality over the course of 10 years (1978–1988) [4]. Standardization may be just as important as the specific clinical practice strategy being implemented. This is important because resuscitation teams frequently deviate from resuscitation algorithms [5]. Finer et al. identified several deviations from resuscitation guidelines, including deep oropharyngeal suctioning, excessive stimulation, poor communication of heart rate, and failure to troubleshoot during bag–mask ventilation [6]. Units in the United Kingdom reported marked variations in practice between units with different designations, suggesting that either the level of care or the experience of clinical staff were factors in the quality of care delivered [7]. Similarly, a national survey in the United Kingdom demonstrated marked variations in delivery room practice; and differences persisted 1 year after publication of revised consensus guidelines [8].

2. Burden and global impact

Adaptation to extra-uterine life occurs during the early postnatal period and is a very high-risk period for premature infants, especially those born extremely preterm. Clinical domains of special interest during the Golden Hours include: delayed clamping of the umbilical cord, appropriate use of supplemental oxygen, non-invasive ventilation, and thermoregulation. Each of these is vitally important components of early postnatal care for the premature infant, and each impacts the others. Multiple studies demonstrate that the complex interplay of interventions in the first few minutes after birth can cause structural changes, trigger inflammatory or pro-oxidant cascades, and predispose premature infants to life-long complications [9]. Therefore, a standardized approach addressing many of these immediate postnatal concerns will likely improve both short and long-term outcomes in extremely premature infants.

An estimated 8 million infants die each year, worldwide. Over half of these deaths occur in the neonatal period, the first 28 days of life. The large majority of infant deaths occur in the first week of life, but the highest risk is on the first day [10]. While developing countries with scarce resources are most affected, the impact of infant and neonatal mortality is significant in industrialized nations as well. In 2010, the United States infant mortality rate was 6.1 infant deaths per 1000 live births, which ranked 26th among similarly industrialized nations. Even after excluding births at less than 24 weeks of gestation, the U.S. infant mortality rate was more than double that of Finland, Sweden and Denmark [11]. Compared to 30 years ago, there has been an overall decrease in infant mortality rates on the first day of life, and this has been attributed largely to advances in delivery room management, non-invasive ventilation, and the use of postnatal surfactant. Nonetheless, infant mortality remains highest on the first day of life, and the first 4 hours is the period of greatest risk [12].

Neonatal mortality continues to be a serious issue, then, even in industrialized nations, and the risk appears to be greatest in the first hours after birth. The risks of adversity are amplified for preterm infants by the unique challenges of transitional physiology, immature adaptive systems, and fragile brain structures. Further, differences in outcomes in similar centers cannot be explained by the characteristics of infants alone, suggesting that differences in care may be responsible for suboptimal outcomes [13]. While this is disturbing, the obvious implication is that interventions aimed at improving early postnatal care can improve outcomes in this high-risk population.

3. The newborn transition to postnatal life

Why is the preterm infant at such great risk? Like infants born at term, the preterm infant must transition from fetal to neonatal life in the first minutes to hours after birth, but the risks that accompany this transition are greater for preterm infants than for infants born at term. Anything that disrupts the normal transition to extrauterine life can have negative effects on physiologic function and outcome. Clearance of lung fluid and lung aeration is perhaps the most important early adaptations to postnatal life. The immature lungs, which are fluid-filled in-utero, must provide gas-exchange immediately after delivery. Similarly, oxygen-delivery to the tissues in-utero is dependent on maternal/placental blood flow, but depends on the infant's immature cardio-vascular system immediately after birth. Once born, the immature myocardium must provide cardiac output in the context of increased systemic vascular resistance and significant circulatory shunts. Various hormonal systems are in transition as well, and organ systems that control thermoregulation, vascular tone, glycemic control and neuroprotection are functionally immature in the preterm newborn.

Immature organ function coupled with the stress of physiologic adaptation to early postnatal life increases the likelihood that the preterm infant will be born physiologically unstable. Indeed, extremely premature infants almost universally require cardio-respiratory support in the first hours to days of life. Mechanical ventilation, continuous positive airway pressure (CPAP) and high levels of oxygen are often needed to stabilize oxygenation and ventilation. This, along with persistent fetal circulatory shunts, frequently manifest as hypoxemia and systemic hypotension in the early postnatal period. The preterm infant is also at significant risk of cold stress. Preterm skin is poorly keratinized and vulnerable to radiant heat and water losses. So while the clinical team is focused on ensuring cardio-respiratory stability and appropriate vascular access, the baby must be kept warm, dry and euglycemic.

The preterm brain is especially vulnerable in the early postnatal period [14, 15]. The periventricular germinal matrix is highly vascular, and susceptible to fluctuations in blood pressure and intravascular volume [16]. Postnatal stress and wide swings in blood pressure increase the risk of severe intraventricular hemorrhage

(IVH) [17, 18]. Oligodendrocyte precursors, present in the primitive white matter, are susceptible to oxidative injury and can have life-long effects on neuromotor function [19]. Moreover, endogenous neuroprotective systems which might otherwise protect the newborn from injury are immature and unable to provide such protections in the extremely preterm neonate [20, 21]. These, and other clinical factors discussed below, explain why the preterm infants is so vulnerable in the early postnatal period, and why the concept of a "Golden Hour" protocol is so important for this high-risk population.

3.1 Early physiologic instability and the risk of subsequent adversities

Physiologic depression is common in the newborn period, and heart rate is the most sensitive and reliable indicator of the response to resuscitative efforts [22, 23]. One of the greatest challenges in neonatal resuscitation, however, is the ability to adequately assess the efficacy of resuscitative efforts. Clinicians are unable to accurately assess chest rise from either the head or side of the resuscitation bed [24, 25], and clinical assessment of heart rate by auscultation or palpation is less accurate than assessments with ECG monitoring [26–28]. Further, even normal healthy newborns may not achieve normal oxygen saturation levels until 5–10 minutes of life [29]. These data, and clinical studies in underdeveloped nations, suggest the importance of the early postnatal clinical assessment [30]. In a clinical study in rural Tanzania, which included all live-born, "lifeless", and stillborn infants, early initiation of basic resuscitation interventions significantly reduced birth-asphyxia related mortality. Mortality increased by 16% for every 30 second delay in initiating positive pressure ventilation (PPV) and by 6% for every minute of PPV required [31, 32]. Preterm infants are at great risk, then, of early postnatal physiologically depression, and there is sufficient evidence that efforts to enhance physiologic stability can improve important outcomes.

The Score for Neonatal Acute Physiology-II (SNAP-II), a validated illness-severity score, derives from clinical data obtained in the first 12 hours after birth [33]. SNAP-II includes six indicators of physiologic instability, among these the lowest recorded blood pressure, the lowest serum pH, the lowest temperature, and the lowest recorded oxygen fraction. In a multi-center epidemiologic study from the Extremely Low Gestational Age Newborn (ELGAN) Study Group, mortality risk was significantly greater among infants with an elevated SNAP-II, and the risk was inversely related to the gestational age at birth [33]. Interestingly, mortality risk persisted even after adjusting for gestational age, suggesting that physiologic instability increases the risk of mortality independent of the risk associated with gestational age. In a separate analysis from the same study cohort, blood gas derangements noted in the first 12 hours after birth were associated with several indicators of inflammation, [34] and these were significantly associated with indicators of brain damage [35]. In a recent publication from the same group, physiologic derangements noted in the first 12 hours were associated with neurocognitive dysfunctions in several testing domains at 10 years of age [36]. Overall, the literature suggests that early postnatal physiologic instability increases the risk of adversity in children born preterm, and efforts to improve physiologic instability could mitigate this risk.

4. Delivery room considerations

Any discussion of Golden Hour strategies begins with delivery room management. It is here that the initial changes in transitional physiology begin, and here that several targeted Golden Hour interventions take place. While only 5–10% of neonates require intervention at birth, neonatal resuscitation is the most common form of resuscitation performed in hospitals worldwide [6]. The Neonatal Resuscitation Program (NRP) exists to guide practitioners in the management of neonates that require help with transitioning immediately after birth. Many institutions employ their own supplementary guidelines and protocols for practice in the delivery room. These focus largely on thermoregulation, advanced non-invasive ventilation techniques, and criteria for administering surfactant. Yet despite the availability of supplementary guidelines, studies have shown that even the most experienced teams will deviate from established guidelines [6]. Like any other skill, neonatal resuscitation and Golden Hour care can be improved with focused practice. Studies have demonstrated that standardized scripts can lead to improvements in care and outcomes. In 2009, Reynolds et al. demonstrated that use of resuscitation checklists, videotaped simulations and team debriefing sessions resulted in improvements in rates of chronic lung disease, intraventricular hemorrhage and retinopathy of prematurity [37].

It is important to recognize that the quality of a resuscitation is only as good as the quality of the resuscitation team. Skilled resuscitation teams improve not only the quality of resuscitation, but the associated outcomes as well. This has been shown specifically with regard to endotracheal intubation [38]. While endotracheal intubation is not unique to NRP or Golden Hour care, this finding suggests that experienced personnel are more successful in high-risk circumstances than less-experienced personnel. Golden Hour care of the extremely preterm infant, especially in the delivery room, should be thought of in the same way. It is not sufficient to advocate for Golden Hour care without first having qualified personnel with the appropriate skillset to perform such care. Moreover, current consensus suggests that interdisciplinary training, team development and the practicing of specific Golden Hour care strategies will not only reduce errors, but improves outcomes [39]. This encompasses strategies such as delivery room simulations with both briefing and de-briefing exercises, as well as content knowledge, technical skills and team building.

4.1 Delayed cord clamping

Delayed cord clamping (DCC), sometimes referred to as placental transfusion, allows the freshly born neonate to remain attached to the placenta, typically for 30–60 seconds. The goal of DCC is to "recapture" as much circulating blood volume from the placental vasculature as possible. This increases the amount of fetal hemoglobin available to the neonate, thus increasing oxygen content, native cardiac output and oxygen delivery. In the premature population, large meta-analyses have demonstrated that DCC has potential benefits for the neonate. A Cochrane analysis published in 2012 concluded that placental transfusion at birth was associated with fewer blood transfusions, better hemodynamic stability in the first few days of life, fewer intraventricular hemorrhages, and fewer cases of necrotizing enterocolitis [40]. Subsequent publications have mostly re-demonstrated similar findings, albeit with differences in certain morbidities and mortality [41]. The theoretical risks of DCC include volume overload and polycythemia, resulting in hyperbilirubinemia, but these risks have yet to be demonstrated in the literature [42].

While there is currently no consensus regarding the use of DCC, it is generally considered safe in term and preterm infants, as long as treatment for hyperbilirubinemia is available. DCC is routinely performed in term neonates, but many institutions also consider DCC for preterm infants born physiologically stable. The randomized control trial by Tarnow-Mordi et al. in 2017 demonstrated no difference in the combined outcome death or major morbidity at 36 weeks in the delayed cord clamping vs. immediate clamping group [43]. Interestingly, this study found a significant decrease in mortality in the delayed clamping group but no difference in the combined outcome after *post hoc* analyses. In preterm infants, it is important to weigh the benefits of delayed cord clamping *versus* those of delaying resuscitation and other Golden Hour measures.

5. Ventilation and oxygenation

Support of newborn's respiratory system is fundamental to Golden Hour principles. In utero, gas exchange occurs at the level of the placenta, but an immense shift in cardiopulmonary physiology occurs at birth. Respiratory distress is common, especially in preterm infants, due to this physiologic transition to postnatal life. The most immediate concern in the delivery room is proper support the respiratory system [2]. A recent update to Neonatal Resuscitation Program (NRP) guidelines highlights several important changes related to respiratory care [44]. These include recommendations on the use of oxygen in the delivery room, guidance on the use of pulse oximetry, and oxygen saturation targets based on the postnatal age in minutes. NRP now advises against routine endotracheal intubation to suction meconium in infants born through meconium-stained amniotic fluids. Revised guidelines suggest prompt intubation of neonates not responding to positive pressure ventilation and for infants requiring chest compressions for cardiovascular depression [45]. Adherence to NRP guidelines is important, as standardization improves care, but adherence to NRP guidelines does not preclude the use of institution-specific Golden Hour practices.

Preterm infants face various challenges in the transition to extra-uterine life. Respiratory drive is frequently depressed, muscles of respiration are weak, chest wall elasticity is high, and surfactant deficiency is common in infants born preterm [9]. This manifests clinically as decreased functional residual capacity (FRC), poor lung fluid clearance and aeration, and ventilation/perfusion (V/Q) mismatch [46]. In addition, the relatively small caliber of the preterm airways leads to greater airway resistance compared to full-term neonates. To overcome this, and to promote lung fluid clearance and expansion, positive end-expiratory pressure (PEEP) are used with great success to support spontaneously breathing preterm infants [47]. The benefits of early CPAP are numerous, including increased FRC, improved ventilation/perfusion matching, and decreased energy expenditure [48]. The need for endotracheal intubation and exogenous surfactant administration reduces, as is the need for mechanical ventilation [2]. While early CPAP has not been shown to reduce bronchopulmonary dysplasia (BPD) rates, it has been shown to reduce other respiratory morbidities at 18–22 months of age [49].

Finally, oxygen should be used judiciously in the delivery room. Avoiding the extremes of both hypoxemia and hyperoxia during the initial phase of resuscitation is crucial. Preterm infants have reduced capacity for mitigating oxidative stress, and are prone to morbidities like BPD, retinopathy of prematurity, intraventricular hemorrhage and necrotizing enterocolitis [2]. For preterm infants, NRP recommends that a pulse oximeter be applied to the right hand or wrist during the start of resuscitation, and that an initial FiO_2 of 0.3–0.4 is reasonable. While optimal goal oxygen saturations based on postnatal age in minutes are not known for extremely premature neonates, the current ranges for term newborns are recommended [2].

6. Glucose homeostasis and early vascular access

A critical component of Golden Hour care is minimizing the maladaptive patterns that accompany the postnatal transition. The premature neonate is ill-equipped to deal with many of these challenges due to immature organ structure and function. One area of particular concern is energy metabolism and glucose homeostasis. Preterm infants are at increased risk of hypoglycemia due to the limited availability of hepatic glycogen stores and brown fat and are at increased risk of hypoglycemia, and its consequences, than are infants born at term gestation.

The developing fetus receives its energy from the placenta in the form of glucose, amino acids, free fatty acids and ketones, with the majority of glucose accretion taking place during the third trimester [50]. Glycogen storage typically begins around 27 weeks' gestation and increases until roughly 36 weeks. Following birth and clamping of the umbilical cord, the glucose concentration decreases to a nadir at about 60 to 90 minutes. Neonates born extremely premature are especially vulnerable during this period as they have limited ability to mobilize glucose, and lack the cerebral defense mechanisms present in term neonates to combat hypoglycemia [6, 51]. Further, the incidence of hypoglycemia is inversely proportional to the gestational age [52]. Prevention of hypoglycemia is therefore an essential component of Golden Hour care for preterm neonates.

Glucose is the primary substrate for cerebral metabolism, and the deleterious short-term effects of neonatal hypoglycemia are well described. Transient hypoglycemia can produce jitteriness, poor feeding, respiratory distress, and in some instances seizures. The risks are greater in premature infants than in term infants. Of greater concern, however, is the potential for long-term neurodevelopmental impairments associated with even transient neonatal hypoglycemia [51, 53, 54]. It is likely that the risks are even greater for sustained or prolonged hypoglycemia. Preterm infants, and infants born small for gestational age, are dependent on exogenous sources of glucose in the early postnatal period. Intravenous access is therefore critical to resuscitative efforts in this population.

Umbilical vein cannulation remains the preferred method of rapid intravenous (IV) access in preterm infants, but a peripheral IV is often adequate. The principle benefits of vascular access are for administering volume resuscitation, maintenance fluids, glucose delivery, and/or medication administration. The presence of a highly skilled, dedicated neonatal resuscitation team is essential for achieving early vascular access and improved outcomes [55].

7. Thermoregulation

Thermoregulation is essential to newborn homeostasis, and this is especially true for the preterm or growth-restricted newborn [56, 57]. NRP guidelines recommend that the temperature of neonates be maintained between 36.5 and 37.5°C after birth through admission and stabilization [58]. Indeed, we have known since 1907 [59] that admission temperature of neonate is a strong predictor of mortality at all gestational ages [60, 61]. Despite these recommendations, it is common for critically ill term and preterm infants to be hypothermic on admission to the NICU; roughly half of preterm infants in the EPICURE Study were admitted to the NICU with a temperature less than 36.5°C [62]. Temperature dysregulation is associated with Apgar scores less than 7, intraventricular hemorrhage, respiratory distress, hypoglycemia, acid–base imbalances, lactic acidosis, and late onset sepsis [58, 63–70].

7.1 Strategies to maintain a thermoneutral environment

Environmental conditions vary significantly from center to center, and even from room to room. One of the most successful interventions is to increase the ambient temperature of the delivery room or operating room to 77–78.8°F (25–26°C) before the delivery occurs [71, 72]. Some authors have described success by increasing the delivery room temperature to 80°F [37]. Since very preterm and very low birthweight infants are at increased risk of hypothermia, various risk-minimization strategies may be needed, including: covering the infant with heat-resistant plastic wrap, covering the infant's head with a cap, use of exothermic mattresses, stabilization under a radiant warmer, and the use of warmed, humidified resuscitation gases [58, 73]. An updated Cochrane analysis suggests that the best approach to maintaining a thermoneutral environment is not yet clear [74]. Techniques recommended for the term newborn are not universally applicable, but may be appropriate for the mid-to-late preterm newborn, including: pre-warming of linens, drying the infant after delivery, removal of wet linens, swaddling, covering the scalp with a hat/cap, and/or placing the infant skin-to-skin based on the stability of the neonate [58, 75].

Serial monitoring of the infant's temperature is imperative, as there is some risk of hyperthermia using the combination of strategies advocated here [76]. In resource-limited settings, or in the absence of the aforementioned supplies, NRP 2015 recommends the use of clean food-grade plastic bag below the level of the neck, and swaddling the infant after drying [58]. Infants who are hypothermic after resuscitation should be rewarmed slowly [58] to avoid complications such as apnea and arrhythmias. Current evidence is insufficient to recommend a preference for either rapid (0.5°C/h or greater) or slow rewarming (less than 0.5°C/h) of unintentionally hypothermic newborns (temperature less than 36°C) at hospital admission. Additional research is needed.

8. Management of infants at-risk for infection

Neonates are vulnerable to infection before, during and after delivery. Worldwide, neonatal infection contributes substantially to neonatal mortality [77–79]. Risk factors for early-onset neonatal sepsis (EOS) include prematurity, immunologic immaturity, maternal Group B streptococcal colonization, prolonged rupture of membranes, and maternal intra-amniotic infection [80]. Chorioamnionitis is a major risk factor for spontaneous preterm birth, especially at early gestational ages, and contributes to prematurity-associated morbidity and mortality. Chorioamnionitis is an independent risk factor for neonatal sepsis, and is associated with white matter damage and cerebral palsy in preterm infants [81]. Late-onset neonatal sepsis has been largely attributed to Gram-positive organisms, including coagulase negative Staphylococci and *Staphylococcus aureus*, and is associated with increased morbidity and mortality among premature infants [80]. Therefore, the timely administration of antibiotics is recommended for at-risk infants.

Early initiation of antibiotics in the first hour of life when sepsis is clinically suspected has been shown to prevent some serious sequelae of early onset sepsis [82–84]. Challenges in establishing intravenous access in very premature neonates may delay the initiation of antibiotics. Application of Golden Hour quality improvement initiatives, including dedicated personnel for placement of vascular access and better communication with pharmacy can lead to improvements in antibiotic initiation time [85].

9. Environment and developmental support systems

Neuronal development begins as early as the 3rd week of gestation and is largely complete by the 20th week of gestation [86]. Neuronal migration begins in early gestation and continues through early childhood. Synaptic pruning, apoptosis, and patterning are important aspects of brain development, and both prenatal and postnatal events play a role in establishing cortical brain development [86]. Biologic and environmental exposures during these critical periods of development can have adverse effects on brain development. Indeed, events or exposures that interfere with these important developmental processes can adversely affect the organization and function of the developing brain [87, 88].

Exposures common to the NICU have been associated with several indicators of abnormal neurologic function, including poor orientation, low tolerance of handling, poor self-regulation, poor reflexes, and abnormalities of tone [89–91]. Conversely, supportive experiences are associated with stronger brain responses in the developing neonate [87]. A NICU environment that provides developmentally-appropriate cares and supports parental involvement and touch likely improves long term outcomes.

Minimizing the frequency of laboratory blood draws, painful procedures, and interruptions to sleep are simple ways of mitigating exposure to stress that can interfere with normal brain growth and development [92]. Noise reduction, human touch, cycling of light, age-appropriate music, and recordings of mother's voice could also be reasonably placed in a Golden Hour protocol to improve the neuro-developmental outcomes of surviving extremely preterm infants [93]. Neonatal programs caring for high-risk preterm infants should include a developmentally-rich and supportive environment as a core clinical domain for the Golden Hours.

10. Quality improvement and sustained outcomes

The International Liaison Committee on Resuscitation (ILCOR), the American Academy of Pediatrics (AAP), and the American Heart Association (AHA) have published guidelines or recommendations on specific resuscitation practices supported by evidence [58]. Translating this evidence and implementing it into practice requires the development of institution-specific guidelines or protocols that standardize as many elements as possible [71].

Low volume centers should develop thresholds or criteria for timely transfer to higher levels of care in addition to developing regionalization of networks of care. Level III/IV centers also should provide leadership and support for regional hospitals and nurseries that make up their referral base, and it is our hope that this publication can be used as a means of enhancing the flow of information to that end [94–96]. Strategies such as the use of checklists, collaboration/teamwork, consistent approach to care, minimizing variation, [37, 97] simulation- based learning with debriefing; [37] development of steps and checklist in Golden Hour protocol, [85] immediate skin to skin in eligible infant [98] have been described in literature to be effective in providing the caregivers ability to remain organized, aware of time management and provide effective Golden Hour resuscitation measures.

Despite the paucity of evidence supporting specific delivery room protocols, the literature favors standardization of as many elements as possible [71]. The introduction of evidence-based delivery room guidelines has been credited with improvements in the quality of care in a variety of clinical settings [4]. Importantly, utilization of standardized protocols has been associated with improvements in morbidity and mortality [99–101]. Ashmeade et al. focused primarily of 4 processes: interdisciplinary team training to improve communication and care in the delivery room, attention to temperature regulation, respiratory support and timely administration of surfactant, and early initiation of dextrose and amino acid infusion [102].

Developing a protocol for any process or improvement requires careful study, inclusion of key stake-holders, thoughtful protocol development and a comprehensive educational process prior to implementation [103]. Quality improvement, however, requires an ongoing evaluation of systems and processes. This continuous cycle of improvement will lead to improvements in teamwork and collaboration, skills and knowledge, consistency of care, and outcomes [104–106]. Consider using this Golden Hour review as a framework for evaluating systems and processes, for developing clinical guidelines or protocols, and for addressing the challenges unique to your institution [107].

10.1 Teamwork and collaboration

Standardized protocols, technical skills, and repeated training are the cornerstones of successful resuscitation. Emerging evidence suggests that human factors, including team interaction, communication and leadership, play a pivotal role in compliance with protocols and the success of resuscitations [108, 109]. One unit described their experience with implementation of Golden Hour protocol that included the use of realistic simulation-based learning, followed by team debriefing sessions as critical pieces of the implementation process [37]. Finer et al., improved their resuscitation outcomes by identifying opportunities and improving team and leader performance [6]. They utilized Crew Resource Management (CRM), a methodology developed for air crews from the late 1970s that evolved from a careful evaluation of the role of human error in air crashes. Communication and team leaders are the primary framework of CRM.

11. Conclusion

Despite advances in medical care, a large number of preterm neonates remain at risk for significant morbidity or mortality. Golden Hour care of the at-risk premature neonate is a philosophical and team-based and highly specialized care that focuses on the first hours and days after birth. It is devised with the understanding that preterm neonates have unique risk factors based on physiology and immature adaptive systems. Key Golden Hour domains include: optimizing delivery room management of ventilation/oxygenation and thermoregulation, early establishment of vascular access, prevention of hypoglycemia, prevention and treatment of infection, and promotion of a developmentally-focused environment that promotes optimal short and long-term outcomes. The available literature supports standardization at the institutional level. In addition, it is critical to have a dedicated team of providers who regularly practice and hone the clinical skills relevant to Golden Hour care. While this discussion can be used as a framework for developing a Golden Hour protocol, each institution, with its own resource limitations and challenges, must devise an approach that captures not only the needs of their patient population, but the knowledge, skills and experience of the team providing care.

Acknowledgments and thanks

The authors would like to thank their patients and their families, from whom we learn every day. Furthermore, the authors would also like to recognize all of the neonatal nurse practitioners, nurses, respiratory therapists, pharmacists, nutritionists, and occupational/physical therapists that work so tirelessly so that we can provide the best care possible for our most vulnerable patients.

Conflict of interest

The authors declared that they have no conflicts of interest to disclose.

Author details

Omid Fathi*, Roopali Bapat, Edward G. Shepherd and John Wells Logan
Division of Neonatology, Department of Pediatrics, Nationwide Children's
Hospital, The Ohio State University College of Medicine, Columbus, OH, USA

*Address all correspondence to: omid.fathi@nationwidechildrens.org

IntechOpen

References

[1] Annibale DJ, Bissinger RL. The Golden Hour. Advances in Neonatal Care. 2010;**10**(5):221-223

[2] Wyckoff MH. Initial resuscitation and stabilization of the periviable neonate: The Golden-Hour approach. Seminars in Perinatology. 2014;**38**(1):12-16

[3] Barrington KJ. Management during the first 72 h of age of the periviable infant: An evidence-based review. Seminars in Perinatology. 2014;**38**(1):17-24

[4] DeMauro SB et al. Improving delivery room management for very preterm infants. Pediatrics. 2013;**132**(4):e1018-e1025

[5] Hunziker S et al. Teamwork and leadership in cardiopulmonary resuscitation. Journal of the American College of Cardiology. 2011;**57**(24):2381-2388

[6] Finer N, Rich W. Neonatal resuscitation for the preterm infant: Evidence versus practice. Journal of Perinatology. 2010;**30**(Suppl):S57-S66

[7] Mann C et al. Marked variation in newborn resuscitation practice: A national survey in the UK. Resuscitation. 2012;**83**(5):607-611

[8] Singh Y, Oddie S. Marked variation in delivery room management in very preterm infants. Resuscitation. 2013;**84**(11):1558-1561

[9] Vento M, Lista G. Managing preterm infants in the first minutes of life. Paediatric Respiratory Reviews. 2015;**16**(3):151-156

[10] Lawn JE, Cousens S, Zupan J. 4 million neonatal deaths: When? Where? Why? Lancet. 2005;**365**(9462):891-900

[11] MacDorman MF et al. International comparisons of infant mortality and related factors: United States and Europe, 2010. National Vital Statistics Reports. 2014;**63**(5):1-6

[12] Auger N, Bilodeau-Bertrand M, Nuyt AM. Dangers of death on the first day of life by the minute. Journal of Perinatology. 2015;**35**(11):958-964

[13] Alleman BW et al. Individual and center-level factors affecting mortality among extremely low birth weight infants. Pediatrics. 2013;**132**(1):e175-e184

[14] Leviton A et al. Systemic inflammation, intraventricular hemorrhage, and white matter injury. Journal of Child Neurology. 2013;**28**(12):1637-1645

[15] Leviton A, Gressens P. Neuronal damage accompanies perinatal white-matter damage. Trends in Neurosciences. 2007;**30**(9):473-478

[16] Ment LR et al. Intraventricular hemorrhage in the preterm neonate: Timing and cerebral blood flow changes. The Journal of Pediatrics. 1984;**104**(3):419-425

[17] Miletin J, Dempsey EM. Low superior vena cava flow on day 1 and adverse outcome in the very low birthweight infant. Archives of Disease in Childhood. Fetal and Neonatal Edition. 2008;**93**(5):F368-F371

[18] Moran M et al. Cerebral tissue oxygenation index and superior vena cava blood flow in the very low birth weight infant. Acta Paediatrica. 2009;**98**(1):43-46

[19] Back SA et al. Maturation-dependent vulnerability of oligodendrocytes to oxidative

stress-induced death caused by glutathione depletion. The Journal of Neuroscience. 1998;**18**(16):6241-6253

[20] Dammann O, Leviton A. Brain damage in preterm newborns: Biological response modification as a strategy to reduce disabilities. The Journal of Pediatrics. 2000;**136**(4):433-438

[21] Dammann O, Leviton A. Brain damage in preterm newborns: Might enhancement of developmentally regulated endogenous protection open a door for prevention? Pediatrics. 1999;**104**(3 Pt 1):541-550

[22] Berger PJ et al. Breathing at birth and the associated blood-gas and Ph changes in the lamb. Respiration Physiology. 1990;**82**(2):251-266

[23] Walker AM et al. Autonomic control of heart-rate differs with Electrocortical activity and chronic hypoxemia in fetal lambs. Journal of Developmental Physiology. 1990;**14**(1):43-48

[24] Schmolzer GM et al. Respiratory monitoring of neonatal resuscitation. Archives of Disease in Childhood. Fetal and Neonatal Edition. 2010;**95**(4):F295-F303

[25] Poulton DA et al. Assessment of chest rise during mask ventilation of preterm infants in the delivery room. Resuscitation. 2011;**82**(2):175-179

[26] Kamlin CO et al. Accuracy of clinical assessment of infant heart rate in the delivery room. Resuscitation. 2006;**71**(3):319-321

[27] O'Donnell CP et al. Interobserver variability of the 5-minute Apgar score. The Journal of Pediatrics. 2006;**149**(4):486-489

[28] Chitkara R et al. The accuracy of human senses in the detection of neonatal heart rate during standardized simulated resuscitation: Implications for delivery of care, training and technology design. Resuscitation. 2013;**84**(3):369-372

[29] Kamlin CO et al. Oxygen saturation in healthy infants immediately after birth. The Journal of Pediatrics. 2006;**148**(5):585-589

[30] Finer N et al. Use of oxygen for resuscitation of the extremely low birth weight infant. Pediatrics. 2010;**125**(2):389-391

[31] Ersdal HL et al. Early initiation of basic resuscitation interventions including face mask ventilation may reduce birth asphyxia related mortality in low-income countries: A prospective descriptive observational study. Resuscitation. 2012;**83**(7):869-873

[32] Ersdal HL et al. Birth asphyxia: A major cause of early neonatal mortality in a Tanzanian rural hospital. Pediatrics. 2012;**129**(5):e1238-e1243

[33] Zupancic JA et al. Revalidation of the score for neonatal acute physiology in the Vermont Oxford Network. Pediatrics. 2007;**119**(1):e156-e163

[34] Leviton A et al. Blood protein concentrations in the first two postnatal weeks associated with early postnatal blood gas derangements among infants born before the 28th week of gestation. The ELGAN Study. Cytokine. 2011;**56**(2):392-398

[35] Leviton A et al. Early blood gas abnormalities and the preterm brain. American Journal of Epidemiology. 2010;**172**(8):907-916

[36] Logan JW et al. Early postnatal illness severity scores predict neurodevelopmental impairments at 10 years of age in children born extremely preterm. Journal of Perinatology. 2017;**37**(5):606-614

[37] Reynolds RD et al. The Golden Hour: Care of the LBW infant during the first hour of life one unit's experience. Neonatal Network. 2009;**28**(4):211-219, quiz 255-8

[38] O'Donnell CP et al. Endotracheal intubation attempts during neonatal resuscitation: Success rates, duration, and adverse effects. Pediatrics. 2006;**117**(1):e16-e21

[39] Perlman JM et al. Neonatal resuscitation: 2010 international consensus on cardiopulmonary resuscitation and emergency cardiovascular care science with treatment recommendations. Pediatrics. 2010;**126**(5):e1319-e1344

[40] Rabe H et al. Effect of timing of umbilical cord clamping and other strategies to influence placental transfusion at preterm birth on maternal and infant outcomes. Cochrane Database of Systematic Reviews;**2012**(8):Cd003248

[41] Fogarty M et al. Delayed vs early umbilical cord clamping for preterm infants: A systematic review and meta-analysis. American Journal of Obstetrics and Gynecology. 2018;**218**(1):1-18

[42] Katheria AC et al. Placental transfusion: A review. Journal of Perinatology. 2017;**37**(2):105-111

[43] Tarnow-Mordi W et al. Delayed versus immediate cord clamping in preterm infants. The New England Journal of Medicine. 2017;**377**(25):2445-2455

[44] Weiner GM, Zaichkin J, editors. Textbook of Neonatal Resuscitation. 7th ed. Elk Grove Village, IL: American Academy of Pediatrics and American Heart Association. 2016

[45] Wyckoff MH et al. Part 13: Neonatal resuscitation: 2015 American Heart Association Guidelines update for cardiopulmonary resuscitation and emergency cardiovascular care. Circulation. 2015;**132**(18 Suppl 2): S543-S560

[46] Hillman NH, Kallapur SG, Jobe AH. Physiology of transition from intrauterine to extrauterine life. Clinics in Perinatology. 2012;**39**(4):769-783

[47] Schmolzer GM et al. Reducing lung injury during neonatal resuscitation of preterm infants. The Journal of Pediatrics. 2008;**153**(6):741-745

[48] Tingay DG et al. Effect of sustained inflation vs. stepwise PEEP strategy at birth on gas exchange and lung mechanics in preterm lambs. Pediatric Research. 2014;**75**(2):288-294

[49] Stevens TP et al. Respiratory outcomes of the surfactant positive pressure and oximetry randomized trial (SUPPORT). The Journal of Pediatrics. 2014;**165**(2):240-249, e4

[50] Castrodale V, Rinehart S. The Golden Hour: Improving the stabilization of the very low birth-weight infant. Advances in Neonatal Care. 2014;**14**(1):9-14, quiz 15-6

[51] Kaiser JR et al. Association between transient newborn hypoglycemia and fourth-grade achievement test proficiency: A population-based study. JAMA Pediatrics. 2015;**169**(10):913-921

[52] Lucas A, Morley R, Cole TJ. Adverse neurodevelopmental outcome of moderate neonatal hypoglycaemia. British Medical Journal. 1988;**297**(6659):1304-1308

[53] Inder T. How low can I go? The impact of hypoglycemia on the immature brain. Pediatrics. 2008;**122**(2):440-441

[54] Salhab WA et al. Initial hypoglycemia and neonatal brain injury in term infants with

severe fetal acidemia. Pediatrics. 2004;**114**(2):361-366

[55] McNamara P, Mak W, Whyte H. Dedicated neonatal retrieval teams improve delivery room resuscitation of outborn premature infants. Journal of Perinatology. 2005;**25**(5):309

[56] Davis PG, Dawson JA. New concepts in neonatal resuscitation. Current Opinion in Pediatrics. 2012;**24**(2):147-153

[57] Narendran V, Hoath SB. Thermal management of the low birth weight infant: A cornerstone of neonatology. The Journal of Pediatrics. 1999;**134**(5):529-531

[58] Wyckoff MH et al. Part 13: Neonatal resuscitation. Circulation. 2015;**132**(18 suppl 2):S543-S560

[59] Budin P. The Nursling: The Feeding and Hygiene of Premature and Full-Term Infants. London, The Caxton Publishing Company; New York, Imperial Publishing Company. 1907

[60] Laptook AR, Salhab W, Bhaskar B. Admission temperature of low birth weight infants: Predictors and associated morbidities. Pediatrics. 2007;**119**(3):e643-e649

[61] Sharma D. Golden Hour of neonatal life: Need of the hour. Maternal Health, Neonatology and Perinatology. 2017;**3**(1):16

[62] Costeloe K et al. The EPICure study: Outcomes to discharge from hospital for infants born at the threshold of viability. Pediatrics. 2000;**106**(4):659-671

[63] Chang H-Y et al. Short-and long-term outcomes in very low birth weight infants with admission hypothermia. PLoS One. 2015;**10**(7):e0131976

[64] Gandy GM et al. Thermal environment and acid-base homeostasis in human infants during the first few hours of life. The Journal of Clinical Investigation. 1964;**43**(4):751-758

[65] García-Muñoz FR, Rivero SR, Siles CQ. Hypothermia risk factors in the very low weight newborn and associated morbidity and mortality in a neonatal care unit. In Anales de Pediatria (Barcelona, Spain: 2003). 2014 2014;**80**(3):144-150

[66] Carroll PD et al. Use of polyethylene bags in extremely low birth weight infant resuscitation for the prevention of hypothermia. The Journal of Reproductive Medicine. 2010;**55**(1-2):9-13

[67] Bartels D et al. Population based study on the outcome of small for gestational age newborns. Archives of Disease in Childhood-Fetal and Neonatal Edition. 2005;**90**(1):F53-F59

[68] Lenclen R et al. Use of a polyethylene bag: A way to improve the thermal environment of the premature newborn at the delivery room. Archives de Pediatrie: Organe Officiel de la Societe Francaise de Pediatrie. 2002;**9**(3):238-244

[69] Mullany LC. Neonatal hypothermia in low-resource settings. In: Semin Perinatol. Elsevier; 2010;**34**(6):426-433

[70] Deshpande S, Platt MW. Association between blood lactate and acid-base status and mortality in ventilated babies. Archives of Disease in Childhood-Fetal and Neonatal Edition. 1997;**76**(1):F15-F20

[71] Wyckoff MH. Initial resuscitation and stabilization of the periviable neonate: the Golden-Hour approach. In: Semin Perinatol. 2014;**38**(1):12-16

[72] Jia Y et al. Effect of delivery room temperature on the admission temperature of premature infants: A randomized controlled trial. Journal of Perinatology. 2013;**33**(4):264

[73] Kattwinkel J et al. Part 15: Neonatal resuscitation. Circulation. 2010;**122** (18 suppl 3):S909-S919

[74] de Almeida MFB et al. Hypothermia and early neonatal mortality in preterm infants. The Journal of Pediatrics. 2014;**164**(2):271-275 e1

[75] Crenshaw JT. Healthy birth practice #6: Keep mother and baby together—It's best for mother, baby, and breastfeeding. The Journal of Perinatal Education. 2014;**23**(4):211

[76] Singh A et al. Improving neonatal unit admission temperatures in preterm babies: Exothermic mattresses, polythene bags or a traditional approach? Journal of Perinatology. 2010;**30**(1):45

[77] Lawn JE et al. 4 million neonatal deaths: When? Where? Why? The Lancet. 2005;**365**(9462):891-900

[78] Lawn JE et al. Every newborn: Progress, priorities, and potential beyond survival. The Lancet. 2014;**384**(9938):189-205

[79] Lozano R et al. Global and regional mortality from 235 causes of death for 20 age groups in 1990 and 2010: A systematic analysis for the global burden of disease study 2010. The Lancet. 2012;**380**(9859):2095-2128

[80] Shane AL, Stoll BJ. Neonatal sepsis: Progress towards improved outcomes. Journal of Infection. 2014;**68**:S24-S32

[81] Thomas W, Speer CP. Chorioamnionitis: Important risk factor or innocent bystander for neonatal outcome? Neonatology. 2011;**99**(3):177-187

[82] Kissoon N, Orr RA, Carcillo JA. Updated American College of Critical Care Medicine—Pediatric advanced life support guidelines for management of pediatric and neonatal septic shock: Relevance to the emergency care clinician. Pediatric Emergency Care. 2010;**26**(11):867-869

[83] Dellinger RP et al. Surviving Sepsis campaign: International guidelines for management of severe sepsis and septic shock, 2012. Intensive Care Medicine. 2013;**39**(2):165-228

[84] El-Wiher N et al. Management and treatment guidelines for sepsis in pediatric patients. The Open Inflammation journal. 2011;**4**(Suppl 1-M11):101

[85] Lambeth TM et al. First Golden Hour of life: A quality improvement initiative. Advances in Neonatal Care. 2016;**16**(4):264-272

[86] Stiles J, Jernigan TL. The basics of brain development. Neuropsychology Review. 2010;**20**(4):327-348

[87] Maitre NL et al. The dual nature of early-life experience on somatosensory processing in the human infant brain. Current Biology. 2017;**27**(7):1048-1054

[88] Noise: A hazard for the fetus and newborn. American Academy of Pediatrics Committee on Environmental Health. Pediatrics. 1997;**100**(4):724-727

[89] Pineda RG et al. Patterns of altered neurobehavior in preterm infants within the neonatal intensive care unit. Journal of Pediatrics. 2013;**162**(3):470

[90] Smith GC et al. Neonatal intensive care unit stress is associated with brain development in preterm infants. Annals of Neurology. 2011;**70**(4):541-549

[91] Symington A, Pinelli J. Developmental care for promoting development and preventing morbidity in preterm infants. Cochrane Database of Systematic Reviews. 2006;2:CD001814

[92] Shepherd EG et al. An interdisciplinary bronchopulmonary dysplasia program is associated with improved neurodevelopmental outcomes and fewer rehospitalizations. Journal of Perinatology. 2012;**32**(1): 33-38

[93] Perlman JM. The genesis of cognitive and behavioral deficits in premature graduates of intensive care. Minerva Pediatrica. 2003;**55**(2):89-101

[94] Lorch SA et al. The differential impact of delivery hospital on the outcomes of premature infants. Pediatrics. 2012;**130**(2):270-278

[95] Phibbs CS et al. Level and volume of neonatal intensive care and mortality in very-low-birth-weight infants. New England Journal of Medicine. 2007;**356**(21):2165-2175

[96] Cifuentes J et al. Mortality in low birth weight infants according to level of neonatal care at hospital of birth. Pediatrics. 2002;**109**(5):745-751

[97] Logan J et al. Congenital diaphragmatic hernia: A systematic review and summary of best-evidence practice strategies. Journal of Perinatology. 2007;**27**(9):535

[98] Neczypor JL, Holley SL. Providing evidence-based care during the Golden Hour. Nursing for Women's Health. 2017;**21**(6):462-472

[99] Coccia C et al. Management of extremely low-birth-weight infants. Acta Paediatrica. 1992;**81**(s382):10-12

[100] Mehler K et al. Outcome of extremely low gestational age newborns after introduction of a revised protocol to assist preterm infants in their transition to extrauterine life. Acta Paediatrica. 2012;**101**(12):1232-1239

[101] Varga P et al. Changes in the outcome for infants, with birth weight under 500 grams, at our department (First Department of Obstetrics and Gynecology, Semmelweis University, Budapest). Orvosi Hetilap. 2015;**156**(10):404-408

[102] Ashmeade TL et al. Outcomes of a neonatal Golden Hour implementation project. American Journal of Medical Quality. 2016;**31**(1):73-80

[103] Sant'Anna G, Keszler M. Developing a neonatal unit ventilation protocol for the preterm baby. Early Human Development. 2012;**88**(12):925-929

[104] Mercer JS et al. Evidence-based practices for the fetal to newborn transition. Journal of Midwifery & Women's Health. 2007;**52**(3):262-272

[105] Morey JC et al. Error reduction and performance improvement in the emergency department through formal teamwork training: Evaluation results of the MedTeams project. Health Services Research. 2002;**37**(6):1553-1581

[106] Helmreich, RL and Schaefer HG, Team Performance in the Operating Room. 1994

[107] Batalden PB, Davidoff F. What Is "Quality Improvement" and how Can it Transform Healthcare? BMJ Quality & Safety. 2007;**16**:2-3

[108] Thomas E et al. Teamwork and quality during neonatal care in the delivery room. Journal of Perinatology. 2006;**26**(3):163

[109] Hunziker S et al. Human factors in resuscitation: Lessons learned from simulator studies. Journal of Emergencies, Trauma, and Shock. 2010;**3**(4):389-394

Chapter 3

Neonatal Bacterial Meningitis

Mehmet Şah İpek

Abstract

Despite improvements in neonatal intensive care, neonatal bacterial meningitis continues to be a serious disease with mortality rates varying between 10 and 15%. Additionally, long-term complications are observed among 20–50% of survivors, depending on time of diagnosis and therapy and virulence of the infecting pathogen. It is more common during the neonatal period than at any other age with the estimated incidence of 0.25 per 1000 live births. The absence of specific clinical presentation makes diagnosis of meningitis more difficult in neonates than in older children. Culture of cerebrospinal fluid is the traditional gold standard for diagnosis of bacterial meningitis, so all newborn infants with proven or suspected sepsis should undergo lumbar puncture. However, deciding when to perform lumbar puncture and interpretation of the results are challenging. Although the pathophysiology of neonatal meningitis is complex and not fully understood, researches on diagnostic and prognostic tools are ongoing. Prevention of neonatal sepsis, early recognition of infants at risk, development of novel, rapid diagnostics and adjunctive therapies, and appropriate and aggressive antimicrobial treatment to sterilize cerebrospinal fluid as soon as possible may prevent the lifelong squeal of bacterial meningitis in newborn infants.

Keywords: neonate, meningitis, diagnosis, treatment, outcome

1. Introduction

Along with the Millennium Development Goals, under-5 mortality rate reduced by an impressive 53% globally, from 1990 until 2015 [1]. Forty-five percent of under-5 mortality now occurs in the first month of life. Besides intrapartum causes and preterm birth complications, infections are one of the leading causes of neonatal deaths [2]. Neonatal sepsis and meningitis are collectively responsible for 6.8% of the global under-5 deaths [3].

Neonatal meningitis is a devastating disease associated with significant mortality and morbidity in both developed and developing countries. The improvements in healthcare delivery systems over the last several decades, especially in developed countries, resulted in a decline in mortality, but the rate of neurological morbidities in infants who survive remains substantial and ranged from 20 to 50% [4–8]. However, the incidence and mortality of neonatal meningitis in developing countries remain unacceptably high, variably reported as 0.8–6.1 per 1000 live births and 40–58%, respectively [7].

Bacterial meningitis is more common in the neonatal period than at any other time, with higher incidence in preterm and chronically hospitalized infants [9–11]. Additionally, the epidemiology of bacterial meningitis, the corresponding pathogens, the immature immune system and its response to infection and outcomes are distinctive to the neonatal period [12, 13]. A cerebral insult related to meningitis has a greater impact on the vulnerable, developing brain, so a younger age during disease is usually associated with a poorer outcome [14]. Therefore, overall improved recognition, evaluation, and aggressive antimicrobial treatment of bacterial meningitis in newborn infants are essential to lead to a reduction in the mortality and the lifelong squeals.

This chapter will focus on the epidemiology, etiology, pathogenesis, diagnosis, treatment, and outcome of neonatal bacterial meningitis.

2. Definition

Meningitis is defined as infection and inflammation of the meninges, subarachnoid space and brain vasculature [15]. Since epidemiology of neonatal meningitis is similar to that of neonatal sepsis, neonatal meningitis is also divided into early-onset and late-onset meningitis, based on timing of infection and presumed mode of transmission [16, 17]. The cutoff for these definitions is variable throughout the literature. Early-onset meningitis is typically defined as meningitis occurring within the first 3 or 7 days after birth, and especially those in the first 2 days after birth reflect vertical transmission of invasive organism from maternal genital tract flora. Late-onset meningitis is usually defined as infection occurring as early as 4 or 8 days after birth and as late as 28 days after birth, and it is attributed to organisms acquired from interaction with the hospital environment or the community [16–18]. In very low-birth weight preterm and high-risk term infants, many of whom have prolonged hospital stays, the description of late-onset meningitis may be applicable until hospital discharge regardless of the age at the time of the infection [16]. The distinction between two patterns is useful to guide therapy. However, this distinction does not necessarily be valid in the developing world, where unsanitary birth practices and newborn care at home or in hospitals confront newborns with the risk of acquiring environmental pathogens at or soon after birth [19, 20].

3. Epidemiology

Worldwide, the incidence of neonatal bacterial meningitis is between 0.22 and 2.66 per 1000 live births. However, the incidence varies by countries of different income levels [11, 20–22].

The incidence of culture-proven neonatal meningitis is estimated between 0.21 and 0.3 per 1000 live births in developed countries [4, 11, 23]. This number is probably underestimated since a lumbar puncture is not performed in up to 50% of infants who were evaluated for sepsis in the intensive care nursery [4], and when it is performed, it may be done after the initiation of antibiotics, likely biasing culture results [4, 24]. The incidence in very-low-birth weight (VLBW) infants may be as high as 1.4%, and about 5% of those with at least one lumbar puncture performed during the hospital stay suffer from late-onset meningitis [25]. Bacterial meningitis occurs in 25% of neonates with bacteremia [17], whereas in LVBW infants with meningitis, the rate of blood culture positivity is as much as 55% [25].

In developed countries, mortality from neonatal meningitis was nearly 50% in the 1970s, and then it has dropped to figures ranging from 10 to 15% [5, 7, 26–29]. However, long-term sequelae rates did not change, with up to 50% of survivors having long-term neurodevelopmental complications [4–8, 27]. In a prospective study including 444 cases of confirmed meningitis during 2001–2007, it was reported that the case fatality for neonatal bacterial meningitis was 13%, but much higher in preterm babies (25%) [29].

It may be difficult to estimate the incidence in developing countries due to under-developed surveillance systems. A few community-based studies published from developing countries tend to reveal higher incidence of neonatal meningitis [20]. In these studies, the incidence of neonatal meningitis in the first week of life ranged from 0.8 to 6.1 per 1000 live births [4, 5, 20]. In developing countries, mortality from neonatal meningitis ranges from 40 to 58% [7]. It is very likely that most of the studies from developing countries have biases in selection of study population, which may have underestimated true incidence rates. Additionally, the lack of laboratory-based confirmation as well as varied clinical criteria and access to health care facilities and limited resources may lead to underreporting in these regions [20].

The most common organisms associated with neonatal meningitis are Group B Streptococcus (GBS), *Escherichia coli*, and *Listeria monocytogenes*, and GBS and *E coli* account for approximately two-thirds of all cases of neonatal meningitis [8, 30]. Thanks to the program consists of identifying pregnant women who are GBS carriers by screening and/or identifying the presence of risk factors that predispose the infants to infection, the incidence of early onset neonatal GBS sepsis in the United States has declined from 1.5 per 1000 live birth to 0.3 per 1000 live births. However, the incidence in late onset neonatal GBS infection appears to remain unchanged or even increasing [30–35]. Additionally, there is an increased incidence of Gram-negative bacteria, specifically antibiotic-resistant *E coli*, in early-onset infection in the preterm and VLBW infants [30].

4. Etiology

The types and distribution of organisms that commonly cause neonatal meningitis depend on age at presentation, location, and gestational age. The distribution of organisms observed in neonatal meningitis is similar to that of neonatal sepsis (**Table 1**) [4, 18, 23]. So, meningitis may be a component of early-onset, late-onset, and nosocomial infection.

The group B streptococcus (especially capsular serotype III) is the major causative pathogen, implicated in up to 50% of cases. Late-onset GBS sepsis is more likely to be complicated by meningitis when compared to early-onset GBS

Causative pathogen
Group B *Streptococcus*
Other streptococci and staphylococci (including especially group D streptococci, *Streptococcus pneumoniae*, *Staphylococcus epidermidis*†, and *Staphylococcus aureus*)
Escherichia coli
Other Gram-negative enteric bacteria (including *Pseudomonas aeruginosa*, *Klebsiella* and *Enterobacter* species, *Proteus* species, *Citrobacter* species, and *Serratia marcescens*)
Others (including *Haemophilus influenzae*, *Salmonella* species, and *Flavobacterium meningosepticum*)
Listeria monocytogenes

For more, see Ref. [18].
†Coagulase-negative staphylococci are particularly common etiologies in very-low-birth-weight infants with late-onset meningitis.

Table 1.
Bacteria causing neonatal meningitis in developed countries.

sepsis [36]. Colonization of the neonate with GBS may be acquired from maternal genital tract during delivery or from nosocomial sources [17]. The attack rate of the colonized newborn is approximately 1%. The risk factors that influence the attack rate include prematurity, dose and virulence of the organism, prolonged duration of ruptured membrane prior to the delivery, and maternal fever during labor [31]. Despite intrapartum antibiotic prophylaxis (IAP) to reduce vertical transmission of GBS infection, not all cases of early-onset GBS are prevented, and GBS continues to be the most common cause of early-onset disease in term neonates [4, 21, 37]. However, it is uncommon in developing countries, even if the prevalence of colonization in women has been reported as high as 22% and implementation of IAP is not possible [16, 38].

Escherichia coli is the second most common pathogen and represents 50% of gram-negative bacteria which account for 30–40% of cases of neonatal meningitis [4, 11, 30]. Most of *E coli* (80%) strains causing meningitis possessed the K1 polysaccharide capsular antigen which inhibits phagocytosis and resists antibody-independent serum bactericidal activity [39, 40]. With the implementation of IAP against GBS, *E Coli* has emerged as the most common cause of early-onset sepsis and meningitis among VLBW infants [41, 42], and it has become the leading cause of sepsis-related mortality in this weight group [43]. Additionally, there is a growing concern on emerging antimicrobial resistance in *E coli* infections [41]. *Klebsiella* spp. are the second most important Gram-negative bacteria causing neonatal meningitis, especially in developing countries [4, 7]. The other Gram-negative organisms less commonly isolated include *Enterobacter* spp., *Pseudomonas aeruginosa*, *Citrobacter* spp., and *Serratia* spp. [17]. *Citrobacter* spp. are usually associated with brain abscesses, emphasizing the importance of brain imaging as part of the evaluation whenever *Citrobacter* is isolated from the CSF [23].

It has been estimated that *Listeria monocytogenes* accounts for approximately 5–7% of cases of neonatal meningitis [5, 28], since the incidence of neonatal *Listeria* infections has decreased substantially in recent years [44]. It continues to be important in contribution to significant morbidity and mortality because of its association with thrombo-encephalitis. Similar to GBS neonatal infections, early-onset Listeria disease is often sepsis whereas late-onset Listeria disease is often meningitis [45]. *Listeria* serotype IVb is responsible for almost all cases of meningitis caused by this organism [46]. *Listeria* may be acquired following placental invasion during pregnancy, passively during the birth process or following horizontal transmission from environmental sources [17, 45].

Coagulase-negative staphylococcus (CNS) and *Staphylococcus aureus* are commonly seen in very premature and high-risk neonates who require prolonged hospitalization, central venous catheters, external devices and ventilator support [5]. Other less common but important pathogens associated with neonatal meningitis include enterococcus, *Streptococcus pneumoniae*, *Neisseria meningitidis*, and *Haemophilus influenzae* [8, 18, 21]. Moreover, there is a wider range of more unusual and potentially antibiotic-resistant organisms causing late-onset meningitis in hospitalized patients [11, 18, 47–49].

5. Pathogenesis

Meningitis most commonly results as a consequence of hematogenous dissemination of bacteria via choroid plexus and cerebral microvasculature into the central nervous system during the course of sepsis [4, 15]. Rarely, meningitis may develop following the spread of an infection in the scalp or skull, and a contamination of open neural tube defect, congenital sinus tract, or ventricular device [4, 18, 50].

The early- and late-onset patterns of the disease have been associated with sepsis during the first month of life, as invasion of the meninges occurs in as many as 25% of infants with bacteremia [23, 50]. So, meningitis and sepsis typically share a common cause and pathogenesis.

Neonates are the most vulnerable of all age groups to infectious pathogens, because of immaturity of the immune system, as well as decreased placental passage of maternal antibodies, especially in preterm infants [16, 37]. All limitations of both initiate and adaptive immunity, decreased inflammatory and immune effector responses, and the deficient expression of complement and of antimicrobial proteins make fetus and neonate, particularly the premature neonate, susceptible to a wide variety of microorganisms [18, 51]. In addition to host susceptibility, obstetric and nursery practices, socioeconomic status, and the health and nutrition of mothers are important in determining neonates at risk for infection, and similarly, in the pathogenesis of neonatal sepsis and meningitis [18, 37].

Initial colonization of the neonate usually occurs in utero from ascending bacteria entering the uterus from vaginal environment after rupture of amniotic membranes [18, 37]. If delivery is delayed, microbial invasion of amniotic fluid may cause an acute inflammation of the fetal membranes, which is defined as chorioamnionitis [18, 37]. Infected amniotic fluid may lead to fetal systemic inflammatory response syndrome, stillbirth, preterm delivery, or neonatal sepsis following invasion of bacteria into the fetus through respiratory tract (fetal breathing), gastrointestinal tract (swallowing), skin, and ear [52]. Additionally, the neonate may be colonized with potentially pathogenic bacteria through the birth canal during delivery. Microorganism acquired by the neonate just before or during birth colonizes the skin and mucosa of multiple sites including the nasopharynx, conjunctivae, oropharynx, umbilical cord, and in the female infant, the external genitalia. Microorganisms can invade through any site where skin or mucosal barrier is disrupted [15, 17]. Bacteria may proliferate at the initial site of attachment without causing serious illness, or then, pass into the subepithelial blood vessel from where they can be transported to other parts of the body including the CNS [15, 18]. Transplacental hematogenous infection is also possible. *Listeria monocytogenes* is usually acquired transplacentally [4, 45]. In rare cases, hematogenous transmission of GBS, *S pneumoniae*, and *N meningitidis* from maternal bacteremia has been reported as causes of early-onset neonatal meningitis [18, 37, 53].

As infants grow up, they are exposed to environmental microorganisms that might be pathogenic to them. Poor hand hygiene among caregivers and hospital personnel, nutritional sources, and contaminated equipment all can transfer microorganism from infected infants to uninfected infants [13, 37, 53]. Most VLBW and high-risk infants have one or more procedures that expose them to risk of infection during their hospital stay. Invasive devices such as venous or arterial catheters, endotracheal tubes, ventricular shunts, urinary catheters, and feeding tubes can insert pathogen into the body of the infant. Parenteral nutrition, exposure to prolonged courses of empiric antibiotics, H_2-receptor blocker or proton pump inhibitor use can also result in increased risk for late-onset infections [13, 18, 37, 54, 55].

Once the bacterium has entered into the systemic circulation, the polysaccharide capsule of the pathogen plays a key role in the survival of the pathogen in the hostile environment of the blood [15, 17, 56]. The polysaccharide capsule mediates resistance to complement-mediated lysis and phagocytosis by polymorphonuclear leukocytes and macrophages [15, 57]. The potential sites for bacteria entering the CNS are the cerebral microvascular endothelium of the arachnoid membrane and the choroid plexus epithelium where capillary endothelial cells are fused along the terminal edge by tight junctions [17]. The attachment of bacteria to microvascular endothelial cells and passage through the blood brain barrier (BBB) are promoted by the interaction of specific bacterial factors with host receptors [57]. To facilitate crossing the BBB, *Streptococcus pneumoniae* interacts with cell wall phosphoryl-choline and platelet activating factor receptor [8]. *Streptococcus agalactiae* uses the lipoprotein laminin-binding protein and K1 *E Coli* express type 1 fimbriae and the OmpA protein to contribute to the bacterium binding to cerebral endothelial cells [57–59]. The bacteria can cross the BBB transcellularly, paracellularly, and in infected phagocytes. Transcellular traversal occurs when the microorganism penetrates the cells without any evidence in the cells or intracellular tight-junction disruption [58]. *Streptococcus pneumoniae*, *Streptococcus agalactiae*, and *E. coli* can all cross the BBB via this mechanism [58]. Paracellular traversal occurs when micro-organism penetrates between barrier cells [17]. *L monocytogenes* crosses the BBB by microbial penetration using transmigration within *L monocytogenes*-infected monocytes or myeloid cells across the BBB by a so-called Trojan horse mechanism [15, 58].

Once bacteria enter the cerebrospinal fluid, they are free to replicate and spread unchecked at least initially, as phagocytes, immunoglobulins, and complement components are excluded by the BBB. This bacterial multiplication goes on until bacteria die following the stationary growth phase or the exposure to the treatment with β-lactams that causes antibiotic-induced bacteriolysis. The subsequent release of subcapsular bacterial products such as peptidoglycan, lipoteichoic acids, lipopro-teins, lipopolysaccharides, and bacterial DNA leads to an increased inflammatory response in the host [15, 59]. Many brain cells including astrocytes, glial cells, endothelial cells, ependymal cells, and resident macrophages can produce pro-inflammatory and anti-inflammatory cytokines in response to bacterial replication and its components [60, 61]. Although this inflammation is needed to eliminate the bacteria and allow the host to recover, it is also a major cause of brain injury in meningitis [11, 61].

Neuronal injury in bacterial meningitis is caused by several mechanisms, which have been identified by experimental studies during the last years [15, 60–62]. Neuronal injury likely results from a combination of the following events: dysfunc-tioning cerebral blood flow (increased BBB permeability, cerebral edema, vasospasm, vasculitis, cerebral venous thrombosis, and systemic hypotension), detrimental effects of inflammatory mediators (e.g., tumor necrosis factor-alpha, interleukin-1, and nitric oxide) and infiltrating cells (leukocytes, macrophages, and microglia), neurotoxicity (free radicals, proteases, and some microbial compounds), increased CSF outflow resistance, and excitatory amino acids, which finally lead to energy failure and cell death executed by caspases [15, 17, 60–63]. The mode of neuronal cell death in different regions of the brain depends on the strength and type of the noxious stimulus and may be a form of apoptotic, necrotic, or hybrid [62, 63]. For example, neuronal cell death occurs mostly as apoptosis in the dentate gyrus of the hippocampal formation, whereas it occurs mostly as necrosis due to focal ischemia in the cortex [15, 62, 63].

6. Risk factors

Since meningitis is most commonly a complication of bacteremia, the risk factors are similar to those that contribute to neonatal sepsis [4–6]. Risk factors for neonatal sepsis include maternal factors, neonatal host factors, and virulence of infecting organism. The most important neonatal factor is prematurity or low birth weight. Small preterm infants have a 3–10 times higher incidence of infection than full-term normal birth weight infants [4–6]. Immaturity of the immune system and diminishing transplacentally acquired maternal immunoglobulins in premature infants contribute to increased risk of infections. Additionally, preterm infants often require prolonged hospital stay and so have one or more procedures such as parenteral nutrition, intubation, and central catheters that place them at risk for infection [18, 37]. Other host factors include hypoxia, acidosis, hyperbilirubinemia, hypothermia, galactosemia, indomethacin, lipid administration, and parenteral iron supplementation [37]. Maternal risk factors include GBS colonization or GBS bacteriuria, prolonged rupture of membranes of 18–24 hours or greater, chorioamnionitis, urinary tract infections, multiple pregnancies, and septic or traumatic delivery [13, 18, 37].

7. Clinical presentation

The earliest signs and symptoms of neonates with meningitis may be subtle and nonspecific, especially more problematic in premature infants [5]. The clinical presentation of neonatal meningitis is similar to those of neonatal sepsis without meningitis. Most commonly reported clinical features include temperature instability (62%), irritability or lethargy (52%), and poor feeding or vomiting (48%) [18]. However, in preterm infants, respiratory decompensation consisting of an increased number of apnea and bradycardia episodes and increased oxygen requirement are prominent clinical signs [50]. Term infants are more likely to have fever (>37.2°C), whereas preterm infants more frequently have hypothermia (<36°C) [64]. Other findings associated with neonatal meningitis include respiratory distress, jaundice, diarrhea and hepatosplenomegaly. However, all these features could not help to establish an early diagnosis of meningitis [18].

Neurologic signs of neonatal meningitis include irritability, alteration in consciousness, poor tone, tremors, seizures, high-pitched cry, twitching of facial or an extremity, focal signs including hemiparesis, gaze deviation, and cranial nerve deficits [4, 18]. Seizures are generally focal and seen in 40% of cases, and considering subtle ones is also possible [5, 18]. Since cranial sutures in the neonate are open and allow for expansion of the intracranial contents and for increasing head size, meningeal signs are not commonly seen. Bulging fontanelle occurs in about 25% of cases and nuchal rigidity in only 15% [28].

Early-onset neonatal infections are generally presented as sepsis or pneumonia, so meningitis is relatively less common. The signs of early-onset infection get to appear within the first 24–48 hours of life in 90% of affected cases [65]. However, late-onset sepsis, in addition to bacteremia, is frequently manifested as focal infections such as meningitis and osteomyelitis resulting from hematogenous seeding [11, 18]. Neonatal meningitis can complicate 14% of episodes of early-onset GBS sepsis and 54% of episodes of late-onset GBS sepsis [36], so the later condition is more likely to have specific signs of meningitis [28].

Lack of data on the timing of onset of features listed above makes it difficult for the early recognition of a baby with meningitis. Additionally, these features are likely to be affected by other factors such as gestational age, partial antibiotic treatment, and postnatal age [6]. Classical meningitic signs such as convulsions, bulging fontanel, altered mental status, and nuchal rigidity are often late findings that are associated with a worse outcome [5, 6]. So, the timing of the onset of clinical features may be crucial for early recognition, prompt management and potentially, better outcome [6]. Although several useful clinical features were defined to predict meningitis in children, the most accurate combination of clinical features to raise or lower suspicion of meningitis is still unclear. Furthermore, small infants presenting nonspecific but concerning features such as fever, lethargy, poor feeding, or irritability, should be approached with a high index of suspicion regardless of how well they appear [66].

Brain abscess, which can be presented by the findings of increased intracranial pressure, focal neurologic deficit, poor clinical response to antibiotic therapy, and new-onset focal seizures, occurs in about 13% of neonates with neonatal meningitis. However, the risk of brain abscess is increased in cases of meningitis caused by *Citrobacter koseri* (up to 75%), *Serratia marcescens*, *Proteus mirabilis*, and *Enterobacter sakazakii*. Therefore, when these pathogens are detected as the cause of the disease, neuroimaging should be performed even with no clinical indication [18, 28].

8. Diagnosis

Since the clinical signs and symptoms are nonspecific and similar to those seen in sepsis, CSF examination via lumbar puncture (LP) is essential to establish the diagnosis of bacterial meningitis and to identify the causative organism with antibiotic susceptibility testing [4]. LP should be performed in all neonates whose blood culture is positive and be considered in all neonates when sepsis is possible. As many as 40% of infants with meningitis who have a gestational age of ≥34 weeks do not have a positive blood culture at the time of their diagnosis [67]. Similarly, among VLBW infants who survived >3 days, one third of cases of meningitis have negative blood cultures [25]. Therefore, if LP is performed based on the presence of blood culture positivity, a significant number of cases of meningitis will be overlooked [11]. This means that if sepsis or meningitis is suspected, performing LP is mandatory.

Debate continues as to whether an LP should be performed on all babies suspected of sepsis or only on symptomatic babies. In the past, the LP had been a routine part of the evaluation of infants suspected of having sepsis, in conjunction with a complete blood cell count and blood cultures [17]. Meningitis in preterm infants with respiratory distress syndrome is unlikely, so an LP is not mandatory unless sepsis is suspected [68, 69]. Similarly, the yield of an LP from babies who are asymptomatic with or without maternal risk factors is likely to be very low [70]. However, during the first week of life, if the blood cultures yield a pathogenic organism or clinical features of sepsis exist, evaluation of CSF should be done [18]. It should be kept in mind that the use of intrapartum antibiotics makes blood culture results unreliable. In every infant older than 1 week, an LP is indicated as a routine part of the work-up for sepsis [17]. Performance of the LP is sometimes delayed due to cardiorespiratory instability, extreme prematurity with the risk of intraventricular hemorrhage, or thrombocytopenia, resulting in delay in diagnosis and prolonged and possibly inappropriate antibiotic use [25]. If it is not possible to perform an LP in the infant with presumed sepsis and meningitis, antimicrobials in doses sufficient for the treatment of meningitis should be initiated immediately following obtaining blood for culture. When the infant is stabilized, even if antibiotic therapy is being taken for several days, LP should be performed. A delayed LP is still likely to show the presence of CSF pleocytosis and abnormal CSF chemistry and thus confirms the diagnosis of meningitis, although CSF culture may be negative [4, 11, 23]. In such cases, real-time polymerase chain reaction (PCR) may have an important role as a better diagnostic tool, although its routine use in the context of neonatal infection is currently limited [11, 71].

Infants with suspected bacterial meningitis or late-onset sepsis should undergo a full laboratory evaluation consisting of a complete blood count with differential, blood culture, a urine analysis and culture (useful only after the third day of life), and lumbar puncture to examine the CSF [50]. Ancillary tests such as complete blood cell count, C-reactive protein, interleukin-6, and procalcitonin have suboptimal sensitivity and specificity for the diagnosis of neonatal sepsis, but these diagnostic tests may be useful in supporting the diagnosis of infection as well as determining the length of therapy when they are serial abnormal and accompanied by clinical features of infection [23, 37, 50].

CSF culture is the gold standard method for diagnosing bacterial meningitis. So, it is important to perform an LP early in the course of illness, ideally before the administration of antibiotic therapy [72]. However, infants may be exposed to intrapartum or empiric antibiotics before performing an LP, making CSF parameters helpful in determining the likelihood of meningitis, because of the possibility of false CSF culture negativity in those with meningitis [4].

9. Examination of cerebrospinal fluid

Although examination of the CSF is highly important in supporting the diagnosis of meningitis, interpretation of CSF findings can be challenging in newborn infants [72]. Values for both the cellular and chemical parameters of CSF are different for neonates than for older infants and children, and also vary according to gestational age, birth weight, and chronologic age (**Table 2**) [73–77]. The cell content and protein concentration in the CSF of a healthy neonate are higher than those of older infants, whereas CSF glucose levels may be as low as 30 mg/dl in

Age [Ref.]	WBC/mm^3	Protein (mg/dL)	Glucose (mg/dL)
Term neonates evaluated in the nursery setting[†] [73]			
≤7 days (n: 130)	Median (IQR): 3 (1–6); 95th percentile: 23	Median (IQR): 78 (60–100); 95th percentile: 137	Median (IQR): 50 (44–56); 5th percentile: 35
8 days to 6 months (n: 140)*	Median (IQR): 2 (1–4); 95th percentile: 32	Median (IQR): 57 (42–77); 95th percentile: 158	Median (IQR): 52 (45–64); 5th percentile: 38
Term neonates evaluated in the emergency department setting[‡]			
≤28 days (n: 3467) [74]	Mean: 5.5; 95th percentile: 16	Mean (±SD): 69.9 (±25.7); upper bound: 127	Mean (±SD): 45.7 (±8.0); lower bound: 25
<28 days (n: 278) [75]	Mean (range): 6.1 (0–18.0)	Mean (range): 75.4 (15.8–131.0)	Mean (range): 45.3 (30.0–61.0)
28–56 days (n: 318) [75]	Mean (range): 3.1 (0–8.5)	Mean (range): 58.9 (5.5–105.5)	Mean (range): 48.0 (30.5–65.5)
Preterm very low birth weight (<1500 g) neonates			
≤7 days (n: 88) [76]	Mean (range): 7.1 (0–30)	Mean (range): 144 (51–270)	Mean (range): 50.4 (11–138)
≤28 days (n: 45) [77]	Mean (range): 5 (0–44)	Mean (range): 148 (54–370)	Mean (range): 67 (33–217)

WBC: white blood cell count; SD: standard deviation; IQR: interquartile range; CSF: cerebrospinal fluid; neonatal intensive care unit; and n: number of cases.
[†]CSF was obtained from infants evaluated for sepsis in the NICU setting.
**In this study, only a small proportion of infants were aged >28 days.*
[‡]CSF was obtained in the emergency department during evaluation for possible infection; infection was excluded by sterile cultures (CSF, blood, and urine). Infants with positive polymerase chain reaction for enterovirus were also excluded.

Table 2.
Characteristics of cerebrospinal fluid in term and preterm neonates without bacterial meningitis.

term infants and as low as 20 mg/dl in preterm infants [77]. CSF protein is higher in preterm versus term infants. Moreover, the values of CSF parameters in neonates with and without confirmed meningitis may overlap [72].

Characteristic CSF findings of neonatal bacterial meningitis include polymorphonuclear pleocytosis, hypoglycorrhachia, and increased protein concentrations [8]. Cerebrospinal fluid white blood cell (WBC) counts of >21 cells/mm^3 in infants with gestational age $\geq$ 34 weeks have a sensitivity and specificity of approximately 80% to suggest confirmed meningitis. However, this cut off may be resulted in a missed diagnosis in 13% of infants with confirmed meningitis, since neonatal meningitis can also occur with normal CSF parameters without bacteremia [4, 67]. If CSF is examined so early, before meninges are not inflamed enough, CSF findings may not be definitive for bacterial meningitis, requiring the repeat LP 24–48 hours later. In a neonate, a CSF WBC count of >20 cells/mm^3 is consistent with meningeal inflammation, and suggests bacterial meningitis [4]. The number of WBCs in the CSF is higher in neonates with meningitis caused by Gram-negative bacteria than those caused by Gram-positive bacteria [78], and can be up to thousands, with predominantly polymorphonuclear leukocytes in the early course of the disease [18, 28]. The level of CSF protein is considered a poor predictor of neonatal meningitis because of considerable overlap of values between infants with and without confirmed meningitis [4, 67]. In general practice, a CSF protein of 170 mg/dl in preterm and > 100 mg/dl in term infants is interpreted in favor of neonatal bacterial meningitis. However, caution should be employed when interpreting CSF parameters in preterm infants [79, 80].

Antibiotic treatment before the LP is a common practice because LPs are not being performed in all cases [5]. When patients with true meningitis are exposed to antibiotics for up to 24–36 hours, CSF WBC values remain elevated without significance. However, CSF protein values decrease but still remain higher than normative values, whereas CSF glucose values show rapid normalization [72, 81]. So, because of limited impact of pretreatment antibiotics on CSF WBC, it does not prevent the diagnosis of meningitis up to 24 hours. Additionally, once CSF is obtained, the sample should be analyzed as soon as possible, otherwise a delay in laboratory analysis may result in the decline in measured WBC [82].

Gram stain of CSF is useful in providing an early presumptive etiologic diagnosis, especially Gram-negative bacteria, since the culture of CSF can take up to 48 hours [6]. Its positivity rates depend on the CSF concentration of bacteria, so the absence of the organism on Gram stain does not exclude meningitis [8]. In cases of meningitis caused by *L. monocytogenes*, Gram stain is frequently negative due to the low number of bacteria in the CSF [17].

Traumatic LP is defined as the presence of blood in the CSF obtained, and occurs very frequently in neonates, with reported incidences ranging from 35 to 46% [72]. This condition makes the interpretation of CSF results more complicated. Adjustment of CSF WBC in traumatic LPs does not improve the diagnosis of neonatal bacterial meningitis, and adjustment can result in loss of sensitivity with marginal gain in specificity [72]. CSF protein may be elevated in the presence of blood contamination from a traumatic LP [83]. It may be useful to repeat the LP 24–48 hours later, so that normal WBC can exclude bacterial meningitis, but frequently it is inconclusive. Neonates in whom the LP is traumatic should be treated with antibiotic presumed meningitis, until results of CSF culture are available.

Among nonculture tests of CSF, the PCR has been useful in the identification of infecting bacteria including *Streptococcus pneumoniae*, *E coli*, GBS, *S aureus*, and *L monocytogenes*, with higher detection rate of any CSF pathogen compared with traditional cultures (72% vs. 48%) in patients with antibiotic administration

[71]. However, the use of PCR is limited to selected cases for now, and before used routinely, requires further researches and institutional facilities [84, 85]. Since PCR neither detects all causes of CNS infection nor provides any information on antimicrobial susceptibility, it should be used in conjunction with standard microbiologic tests. A number of CSF biomarkers such as tumor necrosis factor a, interleukin (IL) 1b, IL-6, IL-8, IL-10, IL-12, IL-17, C-reactive protein, procalcitonin, and lipocalin 2 have been examined for differentiating bacterial meningitis from viral meningitis and noninfectious origins, and the results have been encouraging [8, 86]. However, the validity and use of these biomarkers in clinical practice have been limited, and the interpretation of the results of these assays should be done with caution.

10. Differential diagnosis

Besides sepsis and other specific infections, symptoms and signs may be due to noninfectious conditions such as cardiac, pulmonary, gastrointestinal, and metabolic disorders [11, 18]. Disorders mimicking the neurological features of meningitis include intracranial hemorrhage, ischemic stroke, hypoxic–ischemic encephalopathy, injuries, and inborn errors of metabolism [11, 18]. Conditions where CSF culture is negative despite CSF changes include infectious and non-infectious causes of aseptic meningitis, partially treated bacterial meningitis, parameningeal infected focus such as abscess, and intraventricular hemorrhage. Since some of the pathogens that cause aseptic meningitis have specific therapy, a comprehensive evaluation including viral, anaerobic, mycoplasma, and fungal cultures, antigen detection, PCR, and serology should be performed [18]. Elevated CSF protein values and leukocyte counts and hypoglycorrhachia may develop in preterm infants after intraventricular hemorrhage. Many nonpyogenic congenital infections (toxoplasmosis, cytomegalovirus, herpes simplex virus, and syphilis producing aseptic meningitis) can also produce alterations in CSF protein values and leukocyte counts. [18, 50].

11. Antimicrobial treatment

Eradication of the infecting pathogen from the CSF is entirely dependent on antimicrobial therapy which should be initiated as soon as possible after the evaluation which is suggestive of bacterial meningitis [8]. Since clinical presentation may be subtle and nonspecific and the outcome may be devastating, a low threshold for initiating antimicrobial therapy is necessary without knowledge of the specific pathogen [6]. Decisions on which antibiotics to use empirically are designed to cover the likely pathogens based on the age of the patient (e.g., early-onset meningitis), specific risk factors, data regarding pathogens and their susceptibility within nursery, and the ability to penetrate the CSF [8, 87, 88]. The initial choice of intravenous antibiotics for neonates suspected of having meningitis must cover both Gram-positive and Gram-negative organisms [89]. Efficient elimination of bacteria depends also on the relationship between the concentration of antibiotic in the CSF and the minimal bactericidal concentration (MBC) for the infecting pathogen [17]. Then, antibiotics are modified according to culture and antibiotic susceptibility tests, as indicated.

Initial empirical therapy for early-onset bacterial meningitis must include a combination regimen containing ampicillin and an aminoglycoside (e.g., gentamicin) to cover GBS, *E coli*, and *L monocytogenes*, whereas a regimen including a third-generation cephalosporin (e.g., cefotaxime) is preferred when meningitis resulting from a Gram-negative organism is strongly suspected [8, 18]. This empirical antimicrobial therapy should be continued until the pathogen and its antibiotic susceptibility are identified. Since eradication of Gram-negative bacteria from CSF is often delayed and high rates of ampicillin resistance among E. coli isolates have been reported, cefotaxime is the agent of choice, thanks to its higher CSF bactericidal activity [89, 90]. However, when the use of cefotaxime is routine, rapid emergence of cephalosporin-resistant strains, especially *Enterobacter cloaca*, *Klebsiella pneumoniae*, *Pseudomonas aeruginosa*, *E coli*, and *Serratia* species, can occur (via inducible beta-lactamases), even during therapy [91–94]. It is recommended that such infections should be treated with a carbapenem (usually meropenem), in combination with an aminoglycoside, since carbapenem resistance has recently emerged among Gram-negative bacilli [50, 95, 96]. Therefore, meningitis caused by Gram-negative bacteria need to be closely monitored, which includes repeating LP for documentation of CSF sterility and brain imaging studies with clinical indications [8, 97].

There is a synergy for ampicillin and gentamycin in the treatment of meningitis caused by GBS, and this combination should be continued until sterility of the CSF has been documented [17]. Afterwards, single therapy with penicillin or ampicillin should be used for 14 days [97]. Although GBS is also susceptible to cephalosporins, the use of the narrower agent, like penicillin, will minimize any potential impact on antibiotic resistance among other pathogens [87]. Infection caused by *L monocytogenes* and *Enterococcus* should be treated with ampicillin and gentamycin, since both are resistant to cephalosporins [17, 87]. When the CSF has been sterilized and the patient has improved clinically, ampicillin alone can be used to complete therapy. Because of high rate of ampicillin resistance among *E. coli* and other Gram-negative organisms, a combination of cefotaxime (or ceftazidime in the case of *P. aeruginosa*) and an aminoglycoside, usually gentamicin, is preferable. Once sterility of the CSF is documented, the aminoglycoside can be discontinued and the appropriate beta-lactam should be continued for a minimum of 21 or 14 days after the CSF is sterile, whichever is the longest [17–19, 87, 97].

Initial empirical therapy for late-onset bacterial meningitis usually depends on whether the infection is community or hospital acquired. For babies admitted from home, an empiric antibiotic combination of amoxicillin or ampicillin and cefotaxime is likely to provide excellent cover for possible pathogens, with good CSF penetration [5, 11, 88]. In areas where there are high rates of cephalosporins resistance among *Streptococcus pneumonia,* initial treatment of meningitis may include high doses of third-generation cephalosporins in association with vancomycin before the results of antibiotic susceptibility [98]. Although the implementation of pneumococcal vaccination led to a near disappearance of vaccine serotypes resistant to β-lactams, it also contributed to the emergence of the 19A serotype, which was particularly resistant to antibiotics [98]. Some community-based studies from developing countries have reported increasing resistance, particularly of Gram-negative organism to first-line and even second-line antibiotics [88]. Therefore, in the choice of empirical antibiotics, the resistance pattern of possible pathogens in the community should also be considered.

For babies already in hospital or discharged recently from hospital, initial antimicrobial therapy should be chosen according to the pathogen commonly seen in that particular nursery and their susceptibility pattern [11]. There are various factors that may influence the likely spectrum of causative pathogens, especially their risk of unusual or multidrug resistant bacteria [5, 18]. These include prior exposure to broad-spectrum antibiotics, the presence of central venous lines, ventriculoperitoneal shunt, or ventricular reservoir, parenteral nutrition, and their risk of acquiring infections through nosocomial transmission [5, 55, 99, 100]. Therefore, empirical therapy may include ampicillin (if GBS, *L monocytogenes* or enterococci are suspected), nafcillin, or vancomycin and an aminoglycoside, and cefotaxime, or meropenem, depending on the predominant pathogen seen in the neonatal unit [50, 97]. Meningitis with organisms such as CNS, which is more common in neonates requiring prolonged hospitalization, need for central venous catheters, and surgical manipulations or placement of a ventriculoperitoneal shunt due to intraventricular hemorrhage and hydrocephalus [55, 100], can be treated with nafcillin or vancomycin, assuming that the isolate is susceptible [18, 50, 101]. The duration of therapy is generally 14–21 days after CSF sterilization, with removal of any foreign body if possible [18, 50, 101]. Meropenem is recommended for treatment of neonatal meningitis that is caused by MDR Gram-negative organisms, although it is approved for use only in infants aged older than 3 months for bacterial meningitis or complicated intra-abdominal infections due to limited data on meropenem use in neonates [97, 102]. Metronidazole is the treatment of choice for infection caused by *Bacteroides fragilis* and other anaerobic organisms [18, 50].

The recommended antimicrobial treatment based on causative organism and dosage of common antibiotics used for neonatal meningitis are provided in **Tables 3** and **4** [4, 50, 87, 97, 103, 104].

Although the intraventricular or intrathecal route of administration of antibiotics is able to achieve higher antibiotic concentrations in the CSF and eliminate the bacteria more quickly, intraventricular antibiotics in combination with intravenous antibiotics resulted in a three-fold increased relative risk for mortality compared to standard treatment with intravenous antibiotics alone and should be avoided [105]. However, it remains an option in patients who already have a ventricular drain in place and persistently positive CSF cultures [101].

In the cases of neonates with bacteremia and CSF findings indicative of meningitis with negative CSF culture (obtained before or after antibiotic therapy), the antimicrobial therapy should be continued with meningeal doses as if they have proven bacterial meningitis [97, 106].

The role of routinely repeating CSF evaluation during treatment in a neonate with confirmed meningitis is controversial. Some experts recommended that an LP should be repeated routinely at 48–72 hours after initiation of appropriate antimicrobial therapy to document CSF sterilization, as persistence of positive cultures despite treatment may result in a greater risk of complications and poor outcomes [87, 107]. Gram-positive bacteria usually clear rapidly (within 24–48 hours) from the CSF, whereas Gram-negative bacteria may persist for several days in severe cases [18, 97]. A delayed clearance of a Gram-negative organism may be an indication for antimicrobial resistance and prompts a change in therapy or diagnostic neuroimaging showing a purulent focus of the disease such as an emphysema, obstructive ventriculitis, or brain abscess requiring additional intervention or increased duration of antimicrobial therapy [18, 97, 108]. Additionally, performing repeating LP is also reasonable for discontinuing combination therapy. Delayed sterilization of the CSF is associated with an increased risk of poor outcome [17, 87, 109]. So, a repeat LP may have therapeutic and prognostic significance. Conversely, some experts recommend a repeat LP only if the patient does not exhibit a satisfactory clinical response by 24–72 hours after initiation of antimicrobial therapy or show a complicated clinical course, including seizures, abnormal neuroimaging, or prolonged positive CSF cultures [4, 110]. The decision of whether to perform an LP before completion of therapy in the neonates with meningitis caused by GBS, *L. monocytogenes*, and Gram-negative bacteria can be based on clinical course including seizures, significant hypotension, prolonged positive CSF cultures, and abnormal neuroimaging [50].

Causative organism	Recommended therapy	Comment
Initial therapy, CSF abnormal but organism unknown	Ampicillin IV *and* gentamicin IV, IM *and* cefotaxime IV	Cefotaxime is added if meningitis is suspected or cannot be excluded. Alternatives to ampicillin in nursery-acquired infections: vancomycin or nafcillin. Alternatives to cefotaxime: ceftazidime, cefepime, or meropenem (limit use to multidrug-resistant organisms in nursery (e.g., extended-spectrum b-lactamase-producing organisms).
Bacteroides fragilis spp.	Metronidazole IV	Alternative: meropenem.
Coliform bacteria (*E coli*, *Klebsiella* sp., *Enterobacter* sp., *Citrobacter* sp., and *Serratia* sp.)	Cefotaxime IV, IM, *and* gentamicin	Discontinue gentamicin when clinical and microbiologic response is documented. Alternative: ampicillin if organism is susceptible; meropenem or cefepime for multiresistant organisms. Lumbar intrathecal or intraventricular gentamicin usually not beneficial.
Chryseobacterium meningosepticum	Vancomycin IV *and* rifampin IV, PO	Alternatives: clindamycin and ciprofloxacin
Group A *streptococcus*	Penicillin G *or* ampicillin IV	
Group B *streptococcus*	Ampicillin *or* penicillin G IV *and* gentamicin IV, IM	Discontinue gentamicin when clinical and microbiologic response is documented
Enterococcus spp.	Ampicillin IV, IM, *and* gentamicin IV, IM; for ampicillin-resistant organisms: vancomycin *and* gentamicin	Gentamicin only if synergy documented
Other streptococcal species	Penicillin *or* ampicillin IV, IM	
Gonococcal	Ceftriaxone IV, IM *or* cefotaxime IV, IM	Duration of therapy uncertain (5–10 days?)
Haemophilus influenzae	Cefotaxime IV, IM	Ampicillin if β-lactamase negative
Listeria monocytogenes	Ampicillin IV, IM, *and* gentamicin IV, IM	Gentamicin is synergistic in vitro with ampicillin but can be discontinued when sterilization is achieved
Staphylococcus epidermidis (or any coagulase-negative staphylococci)	Vancomycin IV	Add rifampin if cultures are persistently positive. Alternative: linezolid
Staphylococcus aureus	MSSA: nafcillin IV; MRSA: vancomycin IV	Gentamicin may provide synergy; rifampin if cultures are persistently positive. Nafcillin is superior to vancomycin for treatment of methicillin-sensitive S aureus
Pseudomonas aeruginosa	Ceftazidime IV, IM *and* aminoglycoside IV, IM	Meropenem *or* cefepime are suitable alternatives
Ureaplasma spp.	Doxycycline IV *or* azithromycin IV	Alternatives: ciprofloxacin
Mycoplasma hominis	Clindamycin *or* doxycycline IV	Alternatives: ciprofloxacin

IM, intramuscularly; IV, intravenously; MSSA: methicillin-susceptible S. aureus; MRSA: methicillin-resistant S. aureus; PO, periorally.
†Adapted from Ref. [50].

Table 3.
Recommended antimicrobial treatment for neonatal bacterial meningitis.†

Antibiotic	Susceptible bacteria	Dose per kilogram		Comments
		Body weight ≤ 2000 g	**Body weight > 2000 g**	
Penicillin G	GBS	100,000 U ≤7d old, every 12 h 8–28 d old, every 8 h	100,000 U ≤7 d old, every 8 h 8–28 d old, every 6 h	Monotherapy acceptable if GBS is confirmed by culture and clinical improvement is observed
Ampicillin	GBS *L. monocytogenes Enterococcus* sp.	50 mg ≤7d old, every 12 h 8–28 d old, every 8 h	50 mg ≤7d old, every 12 h 8–28 d old, every 8 h	17–78% of *E. coli* isolates are resistant Poor CNS penetration
Gentamicin/ Amikacin	*E. coli Klebsiella* sp. *Enterobacter* sp. *Pseudomonas* sp. *Citrobacter* sp. *Serratia* sp.	5 mg/15 mg ≤7d old, every 48 h 8–28 d old, every 36 h	4 mg/15 mg ≤7d old, every 24 h 8–28 d old, every 24 h	Poor CNS penetration Synergistic effect with ampicillin in treatment of *L. monocytogenes Pseudomonas* sp. may require combination therapy with a second agent Require therapeutic drug monitoring
Cefotaxime	*E. coli Klebsiella* sp. *Enterobacter* sp. *Citrobacter* sp. *Serratia* sp.	50 mg ≤7d old, every 12 h 8–28 d old, every 8–12 h	50 mg ≤7d old, every 12 h 8–28 d old, every 8 h	Good CNS penetration Used instead of gentamicin in cases of suspected or confirmed meningitis Not active against *L. monocytogenes* or *Enterococcus* sp.
Meropenem	*E. coli Klebsiella* sp. *Enterobacter* sp. *Citrobacter* sp. *Serratia* sp. *Pseudomonas* sp.	40 mg ≤14 d old, every 12 h 14–28 d old, every 8 h	40 mg ≤14 d old, every 8 h 14–28 d old, every 8 h	Good CNS penetration Limit use to multidrug resistant organisms (e.g., extended-spectrum beta-lactamase-producing organisms)
Vancomycin	Coagulase-negative staphylococci *S. aureus Enterococcus* sp.	15 mg ≤7d old, every 24 h 8–28 d old, every 12 h	15 mg ≤7d old, every 12 h 8–28 d old, every 8 h	Variable CNS penetration Effective against methicillin-resistant *S. aureus* Requires therapeutic drug monitoring
Nafcillin	Methicillin-sensitive *S. aureus*	50 mg ≤7d old, every 12 h 8–28 d old, every 8 h	50 mg ≤7d old, every 8 h 8–28 d old, every 6 h	Good CNS penetration Superior to vancomycin for treatment of methicillin-sensitive *S. aureus*

GBS, group B streptococcus; CNS, central nervous system; g, gram; d, day.
†Adapted from Refs. [4, 87, 97, 102, 103].

Table 4.
Dosage of antibacterial drugs commonly used to treat neonatal meningitis.†

12. Neuroimaging

Neuroimaging is recommended to assist in defining the potential complications of neonatal meningitis [50, 87]. Ultrasonography, which is a safe, convenient, and noninvasive method, can be done at bedside early in the course of the disease. It provides rapid and reliable information regarding ventricular size, the presence of hemorrhage, and development of hydrocephalus [111, 112]. It is also useful to detect periventricular white matter injury which may initially be manifested by increased periventricular echogenicity and later by cystic periventricular leukomalacia, ventriculitis, echogenic sulci, and extracerebral fluid collections [113, 114]. Computed tomography is rapid and easy imaging modality, but carries the risk of neonatal brain to radiation. It is useful to provide information on whether the course of meningitis has been complicated by hydrocephalus, brain abscess, or subdural collection. These findings may have a role in decision-making for potential neurosurgical interventions or duration of antimicrobial therapy [28, 87]. Magnetic resonance imaging (MRI) is the best currently available modality for evaluation of the neonatal brain [115]. It provides information on the status of white matter, cortex, subdural and epidural spaces, and even the posterior fossa, when performed either early or late in the course of the disease. It is useful to document the distribution pattern, severity, and complications of the disease [115, 116]. It has also been used in providing the best prognostic information [28]. For these reasons, it is recommended that at least one brain MRI should be performed on every case of neonatal meningitis, especially those caused by organisms that have a propensity for formation of intracranial abscesses [17, 28, 87]. Ideally in all cases, MRI scans must include pre-contrast and post-contrast-enhanced T1-weighted and T2-weighted images in at least two perpendicular planes. Fluid attenuated inversion recovery (FLAIR) sequence and diffusion weighted imaging (DWI) are preferred whenever purulent collections are suspected because of their high sensitivity in showing pus accumulation [115].

13. Adjunctive therapy

Bacterial meningitis in the newborn infant is characterized by high risk of mortality and serious neurological sequelae among most survivors. It is believed that most sequelae occur as a result of neural injury during the acute inflammatory process that characterizes bacterial meningitis. Given that corticosteroids may help attenuate the acute inflammatory process, adjuvant corticosteroid treatment in children with bacterial meningitis may reduce mortality in *S pneumoniae* meningitis but not in *H. influenzae* nor *N. meningitidis* meningitis, and severe hearing loss among children with *H. influenza* meningitis but not among those with meningitis due to non-Haemophilus species [117]. Additionally, these beneficial effects of corticosteroids have been reported in the reports from high-income countries, but not in those from low-income countries, probably due to the types of pathogens prevalent in the developing world, delay in the initiation of appropriate antibiotic treatment, partial treatment involving indiscriminate antibiotic use outside of hospitals, or lack of facilities [7]. A few studies suggest that some reduction in death and hearing loss is evident when adjunctive steroids are used in the treatment of neonatal meningitis, but experimental animal studies reported that adjunctive treatment with corticosteroid is associated with an increase in hippocampal neuronal apoptosis [118]. In conclusion, it should not be used routinely in the treatment of neonatal meningitis due to limited data [119].

Similarly, the limited studies showed that glycerol, when used as osmotic therapy, may reduce neurological deficiency and deafness in adults and children with acute bacterial meningitis [120], but it is not currently recommended in neonates with bacterial meningitis [4].

14. Complications

Short-term neurological complication of neonatal bacterial meningitis includes cerebral edema, increased intracranial pressure, ventriculitis, cerebritis, hydrocephalus, brain abscess, cerebrovascular disease including ischemic arterial stroke and cerebral venous thrombosis, and subdural effusion or empyema [18, 121]. Cerebral edema results from vasogenic changes, cytotoxic cell injury, and occasionally inappropriate antidiuretic hormone secretion [28]. Ventriculitis, which occurs in about 20% of neonates with meningitis caused by Gram-negative organisms, is a result of bacterial entry into the CNS through the choroid plexus [28, 121, 122]. Inflammatory exudate covers the epidermal lining and the choroid plexus, disrupts ependymal lining, and causes subependymal venous thrombosis and eventually necrosis [28]. It is usually associated with obstruction of CSF outflow [121]. Cerebritis results from extension of exudate along perivascular space [18, 28]. Hydrocephalus, which occurs in approximately one-quarter of neonates with meningitis, develops as a result of fibrous inflammatory exudate obstructing CSF flow through the ventricular system or dysfunction of arachnoid villi [18, 28, 122, 123]. Cerebral infarction occurs in approximately 30% of neonates with meningitis and is frequently hemorrhagic [28, 124]. The mechanisms leading to cerebrovascular complications in bacterial meningitis are not completely understood and likely are multifactorial [15, 62]. Brain abscesses, which occur in approximately 10 percent of patients with neonatal meningitis, may result from a hematogenous spread of microorganism into infarcted brain, or by local spread [28, 121]. Subdural effusions occur in approximately 11% of neonates with meningitis and rarely cause clinically significant finding and lead to empyema. [28, 121].

Neonates with bacterial meningitis should be monitored for signs of these complications throughout their treatment. It must be suspected when there is a failure to respond clinically and microbiologically to appropriate antimicrobial therapy, or a focal neurologic deficit, or new-onset seizures, especially focal seizures, or when there are signs of increased intracranial pressure such as bulging fontanelle, accelerated head growth, bradycardia, hypertension, and separation of the cranial sutures [18, 121]. Acute deterioration in an otherwise stable neonate with meningitis can occur if the abscess ruptures into ventricular system or subarachnoid space [28, 121]. In case of suspicion regarding these complications, additional evaluation including neuroimaging studies, neurosurgical consultation, and prolonged duration of antimicrobial treatment may be required.

15. Outcome

In developed countries, the rate of mortality from bacterial meningitis among neonates has declined substantially from nearly 50% in the 1970s to figures currently ranging from 10 to 15% [4, 5, 26–29]. In developing countries, the mortality rate is much higher at 40–58% [7]. Mortality is higher among preterm infants, in cases with meningitis caused by microorganism that causes vasculitis and brain abscess and in late-onset cases [26–29]. Risk factors involved in higher mortality rate and severe disability are low birth weight or prematurity, history of symptoms for >24 hours before admission, leukopenia (<5000/mm^3) and neutropenia (<1000/mm^3), seizures lasting longer than 72 hours, coma, focal neurologic deficits, ventilator support, the need for inotropes, higher CSF protein level, and delayed sterilization of the CSF [4, 5, 24, 26–29, 109, 121–125].

Long-term complications in survivors are mental and motor disabilities including mental retardation, learning disabilities, cerebral palsy, and behavioral problems, seizures, hydrocephalus, language disorders, hearing loss, and impaired visual acuity [4, 5, 14, 27]. Approximately 20% of survivors have severe disability and another 35% have mild to moderate disability [4, 5, 122]. Neonatal meningitis caused by *S. pneumoniae* and Gram-negative bacteria carries a worse prognosis [24, 50, 122, 126]. All infants experienced with bacterial meningitis should be followed long-term for development of neurological sequelae.

16. Prevention

Intrapartum antibiotic prophylaxis for GBS colonized women or based on the presence of clinical risk factors is efficacious against early onset GBS disease but has no impact on late-onset disease, when most GBS meningitis occurs [5, 127]. The incidence of late-onset GBS disease remains unaffected by IAP use [33, 35]. Vaccines against GBS can reduce the number of missed opportunities due to various reasons. So, maternal immunity to the most common serotypes of GBS (serotypes Ia, Ib, and III) can be transferred passively to the fetus and protect against invasive infection in infancy due to covered serotypes [128]. Clinical trials of a trivalent GBS vaccine are encouraging in this regard. In the case of pneumococcal meningitis, the 10- and 13-valent conjugate vaccines may be protective for infants aged <3 months [5].

The prevention of the spread of the pathogens responsible for neonatal sepsis and meningitis also has an impact on disease burden [6]. Several interventions, which can be introduced at the community level, with prevention strategies applied during the antenatal, intrapartum, and early neonatal period, will reduce the number of early-onset diseases [16, 129]. Prevention of nosocomial infections is based on strategies that aim to limit susceptibility to infections by enhancing host defenses, interrupting transmission of organisms by healthcare workers, and by promoting the judicious use of antimicrobials [130].

17. Summary

Bacterial meningitis is associated with significant morbidity and mortality in the neonatal population. Although overall incidence and mortality have declined over the last several decades, morbidity associated with neonatal meningitis remains unchanged. Prompt diagnosis and treatment are mandatory to improve both short- and long-term outcomes. CSF culture obtained via LP is the gold-standard method for the diagnosis of meningitis, which is the key to rapid institution of effective antimicrobial therapy. Prevention strategies, adjunctive therapies, improved diagnostic strategies, and development of vaccines may further reduce the burden of this devastating disease.

Conflict of interest

The author declares no conflicts of interest.

Neonatal Bacterial Meningitis
DOI: http://dx.doi.org/10.5772/intechopen.87118

Author details

Mehmet Şah İpek
Division of Neonatology, Department of Pediatrics, Memorial Dicle Hospital,
Diyarbakir, Turkey

*Address all correspondence to: md.msipek@yahoo.com

IntechOpen

References

[1] GBD 2015 Child Mortality Collaborators. Global, regional, national, and selected subnational levels of stillbirths, neonatal, infant, and under-5 mortality, 1980-2015: A systematic analysis for the Global Burden of Disease Study 2015. Lancet. 2016;**388**:1725-1774

[2] Lawn J, Blencowe H, Oza S, et al. Every newborn: Progress, priorities, and potential beyond survival. Lancet. 2014;**384**:189-205

[3] Liu L, Oza S, Hogan D, et al. Global, regional, and national causes of under-5 mortality in 2000-15: An updated systematic analysis with implications for the sustainable development goals. Lancet. 2016;**388**:3027-3035

[4] Ku LC, Boggess KA, Cohen-Wolkowiez M. Bacterial meningitis in infants. Clinics in Perinatology. 2015;**42**:29-45

[5] Heath PT, Okike IO, Oeser C. Neonatal meningitis: Can we do better? Advances in Experimental Medicine and Biology. 2011;**719**:11-24

[6] Galiza EP, Heath PT. Improving the outcome of neonatal meningitis. Current Opinion in Infectious Diseases. 2009;**22**:229-234

[7] Furyk JS, Swann O, Molyneux E. Systematic review: Neonatal meningitis in the developing world. Tropical Medicine & International Health. 2011;**16**:672-679

[8] Kim KS. Neonatal bacterial meningitis. NeoReviews. 2015;**16**:e535

[9] Wenger JD, Hightower AW, Facklam RR, et al. Bacterial meningitis in the United States, 1986: Report of a multistate surveillance study. The bacterial meningitis study group.

The Journal of Infectious Diseases. 1990;**162**:1316-1323

[10] de Louvois J, Blackbourn J, Hurley R, et al. Infantile meningitis in England and Wales: A two year study. Archives of Disease in Childhood. 1991;**66**:603-607

[11] Heath PT, Okike IO. Neonatal bacterial meningitis: An update. Paediatrics and Child Health. 2010;**20**:526-530

[12] Cantey JB, Milstone AM. Bloodstream infections: Epidemiology and resistance. Clinics in Perinatology. 2015;**42**:1-16

[13] Camacho-Gonzalez A, Spearman PW, Stoll BJ. Neonatal infectious diseases: Evaluation of neonatal sepsis. Pediatric Clinics of North America. 2013;**60**:367-389

[14] Anderson V, Anderson P, Grimwood K, et al. Cognitive and executive function 12 years after childhood bacterial meningitis: Effect of acute neurologic complications and age of onset. Journal of Pediatric Psychology. 2004;**29**:67-81

[15] Grandgirard D, Leib SL. Meningitis in neonates: Bench to bedside. Clinics in Perinatology. 2010;**37**:655-676

[16] Ganatra HA, Stoll BJ, Zaidi AK. International perspective on early-onset neonatal sepsis. Clinics in Perinatology. 2010;**37**:501-523

[17] Polin RA, Harris MC. Neonatal bacterial meningitis. Seminars in Neonatology. 2001;**6**:157-172

[18] Nizet V, Klein JO. Bacterial sepsis and meningitis. In: Wilson CB, Nizet V, Maldonado Y, editors. Remington and Klein's Infectious Diseases of the Fetus and Newborn. 8th ed. Philadelphia: Elsevier Saunders; 2016. pp. 217-271

[19] Zaidi AK, Huskins WC, Thaver D, et al. Hospital-acquired neonatal infections in developing countries. Lancet. 2005;**365**:1175-1188

[20] Thaver D, Zaidi AK. Burden of neonatal infections in developing countries: A review of evidence from community-based studies. The Pediatric Infectious Disease Journal. 2009;**28**:S3-S9

[21] Okike IO, Johnson AP, Henderson KL, et al. Incidence, aetiology and outcome of bacterial meningitis in infants aged <90 days in the UK and Republic of Ireland: Prospective, enhanced, national population-based surveillance. Clinical Infectious Diseases. 2014;**59**:e150-e157

[22] Kavuncuoglu S, Gursoy S, Turel O, et al. Neonatal bacterial meningitis in Turkey: Epidemiology, risk factors, and prognosis. Journal of Infection in Developing Countries. 2013;**7**:73-81

[23] Leonard EG, Dobbs K. Postnatal bacterial infections. In: Martin RJ, Fanaroff AA, Walsh MC, editors. Fanaroff and Martin's Neonatal-Perinatal Medicine: Diseases of the Fetus and Infant. 10th ed. Philadelphia: Saunders/Elsevier; 2015. pp. 734-750

[24] May M, Daley AJ, Donath S, et al. Early onset neonatal meningitis in Australia and New Zealand: 1992-2002. Archives of Disease in Childhood. Fetal and Neonatal Edition. 2005;**90**:F324-F327

[25] Stoll BJ, Hansen N, Fanaroff AA, et al. To tap or not to tap: High likelihood of meningitis without sepsis among very low birth weight infants. Pediatrics. 2004;**113**:1181-1186

[26] Harvey D, Holt DE, Bedford H. Bacterial meningitis in the newborn: A prospective study of mortality and morbidity. Seminars in Perinatology. 1999;**23**:218

[27] de Louvois J, Halket S, Harvey D. Neonatal meningitis in England and Wales: Sequelae at 5 years of age. European Journal of Pediatrics. 2005;**164**:730

[28] Baud O, Aujard Y. Neonatal bacterial meningitis. Handbook of Clinical Neurology. 2013;**112**:1109-1113

[29] Gaschignard J, Levy C, Romain O, et al. Neonatal bacterial meningitis, 444 cases in 7 years. The Pediatric Infectious Disease Journal. 2011;**30**:212-217

[30] Stoll BJ, Hansen NI, Sanchez PJ, et al. Early onset neonatal sepsis: The burden of group B streptococcal and *E. coli* disease continues. Pediatrics. 2011;**127**:817-826

[31] Oh W. Early onset neonatal group B streptococcal sepsis. American Journal of Perinatology. 2013;**30**:143-147

[32] Okike IO, Ribeiro S, Ramsay ME, et al. Trends in bacterial, mycobacterial, and fungal meningitis in England and Wales 2004-11: An observational study. The Lancet Infectious Diseases. 2014;**14**:301-307

[33] Berardi A, Rossi C, Lugli L, et al. Group B streptococcus late-onset disease: 2003-2010. Pediatrics. 2013;**131**:e361-e368

[34] Lamagni TL, Keshishian C, Efstratiou A, et al. Emerging trends in the epidemiology of invasive group B streptococcal disease in England and Wales, 1991-2010. Clinical Infectious Diseases. 2013;**57**:682-688

[35] Schrag SJ, Verani JR. Intrapartum antibiotic prophylaxis for the prevention of perinatal group B streptococcal disease: Experience in the United States and implications for a potential group B streptococcal vaccine. Vaccine. 2013;**31**:d20-d26

[36] Ansong AK, Smith PB, Benjamin DK, et al. Group B streptococcal

meningitis: Cerebrospinal fluid parameters in the era of intrapartum antibiotic prophylaxis. Early Human Development. 2009;**85**:S5-S7

[37] Shane AL, Sánchez PJ, Stoll BJ. Neonatal sepsis. Lancet. 2017;**390**:1770-1780

[38] Vergnano S, Sharland M, Kazembe P, et al. Neonatal sepsis: An international perspective. Archives of Disease in Childhood. Fetal and Neonatal Edition. 2005;**90**:F220-F224

[39] Sarff LD, McCracken GH Jr, Scheffen MS, et al. Epidermiology of *Escherichia coli* K1 in healthy and diseased newborns. Lancet. 1975;**1**:1099-1104

[40] Bingen E, Bonacorsi S, Brahimi N, et al. Virulence patterns of *Escherichia coli* and K1 strains associated with neonatal meningitis. Journal of Clinical Microbiology. 1997;**35**:2981-2982

[41] Bizzarro, Dembry LM, Baltimore RS, et al. Changing patterns in neonatal *Escherichia coli* sepsis and ampicillin resistance in the era of intrapartum antibiotic prophylaxis. Pediatrics. 2008;**121**:689-696

[42] Stoll BJ, Hansen NI, Higgins RD, et al. Very low birth weight preterm infants with early onset neonatal sepsis: The predominance of gram-negative infections continues in the National Institute of child health and human development neonatal research network, 2002-2003. The Pediatric Infectious Disease Journal. 2005;**24**:635-639

[43] Weston EJ, Pondo T, Lewis MM, et al. The burden of invasive early-onset neonatal sepsis in the United States, 2005-2008. The Pediatric Infectious Disease Journal. 2011;**30**:937-941

[44] Lee B, Newland JG, Jhaveri R. Reductions in neonatal listeriosis:

"Collateral benefit" of group B streptococcal prophylaxis? The Journal of Infection. 2016;**72**:317-323

[45] McKinney JS. Listeria infections in neonates. NeoReviews. 2016;**17**:e515-e520

[46] Smith B. Listeria monocytogenes: Maternal-foetal infections in Denmark 1994-2005. Scandinavian Journal of Infectious Diseases. 2009;**41**:21-25

[47] Giacoia GP. Uncommon pathogens in newborn infants. Journal of Perinatology. 1994;**14**:134-144

[48] İpek MS, Ozbek E, Guldemir D, et al. Neonatal meningitis caused by Actinomyces: A case report of the most probably new strain. Journal of Pediatric Infectious Diseases. 2017;**12**:138-141

[49] Uchida Y, Morita H, Adachi S, et al. Bacterial meningitis and septicemia of neonate due to *Lactococcus lactis*. Pediatrics International. 2011 Feb;**53**:119-120

[50] Kaufman D, Zanelli S, Sánchez PJ. Neonatal meningitis: Current treatment options. In: Perlman JM, editor. Neurology: Neonatology Questions and Controversies. 3th ed. Philadelphia: Elsevier Saunders; 2019. pp. 187-205

[51] Wynn JL, Levy O. Role of innate host defenses in susceptibility to early-onset neonatal sepsis. Clinics in Perinatology. 2010;**37**:307-337

[52] Kim CJ, Romero R, Chaemsaithong P, et al. Acute chorioamnionitis and funisitis: Definition, pathologic features, and clinical significance. American Journal of Obstetrics and Gynecology. 2015;**213**:S29-S52

[53] Hughes BR, Mercer JL, Gosbel LB. Neonatal pneumococcal sepsis in association with fatal maternal pneumococcal sepsis. The Australian &

New Zealand Journal of Obstetrics & Gynaecology. 2001;**41**:457-458

[54] Clark R, Powers R, White R, et al. Nosocomial infection in the NICU: A medical complication or unavoidable problem? Journal of Perinatology. 2004;**24**:382-388

[55] Stoll BJ, Hansen N, Fanaroff AA, et al. Late-onset sepsis in very low birth weight neonates: The experience of the NICHD neonatal research network. Pediatrics. 2002;**110**:285-291

[56] Kim KS. Acute bacterial meningitis in infants and children. The Lancet Infectious Diseases. 2010;**10**:32-42

[57] Kim KS, Itabashi H, Gemski P, et al. The K1 capsule is the critical determinant in the development of *Escherichia coli* meningitis in the rat. The Journal of Clinical Investigation. 1992;**90**:897-905

[58] Kim KS. Mechanisms of microbial traversal of the blood-brain barrier. Nature Reviews. Microbiology. 2008;**6**(8):625-634

[59] Tenenbaum T, Spellerberg B, Adam R, et al. *Streptococcus agalactiae* invasion of human brain microvascular endothelial cells is promoted by the laminin-binding protein Lmb. Microbes and Infection. 2007;**9**:714-720

[60] Barichello T, Fagundes GD, Generoso JS, et al. Pathophysiology of neonatal acute bacterial meningitis. Journal of Medical Microbiology. 2013;**62**:1781-1789

[61] Tauber MG, Moser B. Cytokines and chemokines in meningeal inflammation: Biology and clinical implications. Clinical Infectious Diseases. 1999;**28**:1-12

[62] Gerber J, Nau R. Mechanisms of injury in bacterial meningitis. Current Opinion in Neurology. 2010;**23**:312-318

[63] Liechti FD, Grandgirard D, Leib SL. Bacterial meningitis: Insights into pathogenesis and evaluation of new treatment options: A perspective from experimental studies. Future Microbiology. 2015;**10**:1195-1213

[64] Weisman LE, Stoll BJ, Cruess DF, et al. Early-onset group B streptococcal sepsis: A current assessment. The Journal of Pediatrics. 1992;**121**:428-433

[65] Escobar GJ, Puopolo KM, Wi S, Turk BJ, et al. Stratification of risk of early-onset sepsis in newborns ≥34 weeks' gestation. Pediatrics. 2014;**133**:30-36

[66] Curtis S, Stobart K, Vandermeer B, et al. Clinical features suggestive of meningitis in children: A systematic review of prospective data. Pediatrics. 2010;**126**:952-960

[67] Garges HP, Moody MA, Cotten CM, et al. Neonatal meningitis: What is the correlation among cerebrospinal fluid cultures, blood cultures, and cerebrospinal fluid parameters? Pediatrics. 2006;**117**:1094-1100

[68] Hendricks-Muñoz KD, Shapiro DL. The role of the lumbar puncture in the admission sepsis evaluation of the premature infant. Journal of Perinatology. 1990;**10**:60-64

[69] Eldadah M, Frenkel LD, Hiatt IM, et al. Evaluation of routine lumbar punctures in newborn infants with respiratory distress syndrome. The Pediatric Infectious Disease Journal. 1987;**6**:243-246

[70] Fielkow S, Reuter S, Gotoff SP. Cerebrospinal fluid examination in symptom-free infants with risk factors for infection. The Journal of Pediatrics. 1991;**119**:971-973

[71] Chiba N, Murayama SY, Morozumi M, et al. Rapid detection of eight causative pathogens for the diagnosis of bacterial meningitis by

real-time PCR. Journal of Infection and Chemotherapy. 2009;**15**:92-98

[72] Srinivasan L, Harris MC, Shah SS. Lumbar puncture in the neonate: Challenges in decision making and interpretation. Seminars in Perinatology. 2012;**36**:445-453

[73] Srinivasan L, Shah SS, Padula MA, et al. Cerebrospinal fluid reference ranges in term and preterm infants in the neonatal intensive care unit. The Journal of Pediatrics. 2012;**161**:729-734

[74] Thomson J, Sucharew H, Cruz AT, et al. Cerebrospinal fluid reference values for young infants undergoing lumbar puncture. Pediatrics. 2018;**141**. pii: e20173405

[75] Byington CL, Kendrick J, Sheng X. Normative cerebrospinal fluid profiles in febrile infants. The Journal of Pediatrics. 2011;**158**:130-134

[76] Mhanna MJ, Alesseh H, Gori A, et al. Cerebrospinal fluid values in very low birth weight infants with suspected sepsis at different ages. Pediatric Critical Care Medicine. 2008;**9**:294-298

[77] Rodriguez AF, Kaplan SL, Mason EO. Cerebrospinal fluid values in the very low birth weight infant. The Journal of Pediatrics. 1990;**116**:971-974

[78] Smith PB, Cotten CM, Garges HP, et al. A comparison of neonatal Gram-negative rod and Gram-positive cocci meningitis. Journal of Perinatology. 2006;**26**:111-114

[79] Shah SS, Ebberson J, Kestenbaum LA, et al. Age-specific reference values for cerebrospinal fluid protein concentration in neonates and young infants. Journal of Hospital Medicine. 2011;**6**:22-27

[80] Smith PB, Garges HP, Cotton CM, et al. Meningitis in preterm neonates: Importance of cerebrospinal fluid parameters. American Journal of Perinatology. 2008;**25**:421-416

[81] Nigrovic LE, Malley R, Macias CG, et al. Effect of antibiotic pretreatment on cerebrospinal fluid profiles of children with bacterial meningitis. Pediatrics. 2008;**122**:726-730

[82] Rajesh NT, Dutta S, Prasad R, Narang A. Effect of delay in analysis on neonatal cerebrospinal fluid parameters. Archives of Disease in Childhood. Fetal and Neonatal Edition. 2010;**95**:F25-F29

[83] Hines EM, Nigrovic LE, Neuman MI, et al. Adjustment of cerebrospinal fluid protein for red blood cells in neonates and young infants. Journal of Hospital Medicine. 2012;**7**:325-328

[84] Liu CL, Ai HW, Wang WP, et al. Comparison of 16S rRNA gene PCR and blood culture for diagnosis of neonatal sepsis. Archives de Pédiatrie. 2014;**21**:162-169

[85] El Gawhary S, El-Anany M, Hassan R, et al. The role of 16S rRNA gene sequencing in confirmation of suspected neonatal sepsis. Journal of Tropical Pediatrics. 2016;**62**:75-80

[86] Gordon SM, Srinivasan L, Harris MC. Neonatal meningitis: Overcoming challenges in diagnosis, prognosis, and treatment with omics. Frontiers in Pediatrics. 2017;**5**:139

[87] Heath PT, Nik Yusoff NK, Baker CJ. Neonatal meningitis. Archives of Disease in Childhood. Fetal and Neonatal Edition. 2003;**88**:F173-F178

[88] Zaidi AK, Thaver D, Ali SA, et al. Pathogens associated with sepsis in newborns and young infants in developing countries. The Pediatric Infectious Disease Journal. 2009;**28**:S10-S18

[89] Quagliarello VJ, Scheld WM. Treatment of bacterial meningitis.

The New England Journal of Medicine. 1997;**336**:708-716

[90] Cherubin CE, Eng RH, Norrby R, et al. Penetration of newer cephalosporins into cerebrospinal fluid. Reviews of Infectious Diseases. 1989;**11**:526-548

[91] Wong-Beringer A, Hindler J, Loeloff M, et al. Molecular correlation for the treatment outcomes in bloodstream infections caused by *Escherichia coli* and *Klebsiella pneumoniae* with reduced susceptibility to ceftazidime. Clinical Infectious Diseases. 2002;**34**:135-146

[92] Patterson JE. Extended spectrum beta-lactamases: A therapeutic dilemma. The Pediatric Infectious Disease Journal. 2002;**21**:957-959

[93] Shah AA, Hasan F, Ahmed S, et al. Characteristics, epidemiology and clinical importance of emerging strains of Gram-negative bacilli producing extended-spectrum beta-lactamases. Research in Microbiology. 2004;**155**:409-421

[94] Thaver D, Ali SA, Zaidi AK. Antimicrobial resistance among neonatal pathogens in developing countries. The Pediatric Infectious Disease Journal. 2009;**28**:S19-S21

[95] Folgori L, Bielicki J, Heath PT, et al. Antimicrobial-resistant Gram-negative infections in neonates: Burden of disease and challenges in treatment. Current Opinion in Infectious Diseases. 2017;**30**:281-288

[96] İpek MS, Aktar F, Okur N, et al. Colistin use in critically ill neonates: A case-control study. Pediatrics and Neonatology. 2017;**58**:490-496

[97] Edwards MS, Baker CJ. Bacterial meningitis in the neonate: Treatment and outcome. In: Kaplan SL, Weisman LE, editors. UpToDate. Waltam, MA: UpToDate Inc. Available from: https://www.uptodate.com [Accessed: September 15, 2018]

[98] Cohen R, Raymond J, Hees L, et al. Bacterial meningitis antibiotic treatment. Archives de Pédiatrie. 2017;**24**:S42-S45

[99] Gray JW. Surveillance of infection in neonatal intensive care units. Early Human Development. 2007;**83**:157-163

[100] Marchant EA, Boyce GK, Sadarangani M, et al. Neonatal sepsis due to coagulase-negative staphylococci. Clinical & Developmental Immunology. 2013;**2013**:586076

[101] Arnell K, Enblad P, Wester T, et al. Treatment of cerebrospinal fluid shunt infections in children using systemic and intraventricular antibiotic therapy in combination with externalization of the ventricular catheter: Efficacy in 34 consecutively treated infections. Journal of Neurosurgery. 2007;**107**:213-219

[102] Pacifici GM, Allegaert K. Clinical pharmacology of carbapenems in neonates. Journal of Chemotherapy. 2014;**26**:67-73

[103] Schleiss MR. Principles of antibacterial therapy. In: Kliegman RM, Stanton B, Geme JS, Schor NF, editors. Nelson Textbook of Pediatrics. 20th ed. Philadelphia: Elsevier Saunder; 2016. pp. 1298-1315.e1

[104] American Academy of Pediatrics. Red Book: Report of the Committee on Infectious Diseases. Committee on Infectious Diseases; 2015. pp. 881-883

[105] Shah SS, Ohlsson A, Shah VS. Intraventricular antibiotics for bacterial meningitis in neonates. Cochrane Database of Systematic Reviews. 2012;**7**:CD004496

[106] Huang FK, Chen HL, Yang PH, et al. Bird's eye view of a neonatologist: Clinical approach to emergency

neonatal infection. Pediatrics and Neonatology. 2016;57:167-173

[107] Lebel MH, McCracken GH Jr. Delayed cerebrospinal fluid sterilization and adverse outcome of bacterial meningitis in infants and children. Pediatrics. 1989;83:161-167

[108] Tunkel AR, Scheld WM. Issues in the management of bacterial meningitis. American Family Physician. 1997;56:1355-1362

[109] Greenberg RG, Benjamin DK Jr, Cohen-Wolkowiez M, et al. Repeat lumbar punctures in infants with meningitis in the neonatal intensive care unit. Journal of Perinatology. 2011;31:425-429

[110] Agarwal R, Emmerson AJ. Should repeat lumbar punctures be routinely done in neonates with bacterial meningitis? Results of a survey into clinical practice. Archives of Disease in Childhood. 2001;84:451-452

[111] Perlman JM, Rollins N, Sanchez PJ. Late-onset meningitis in sick, very-low-birth-weight infants. Clinical and sonographic observations. American Journal of Diseases of Children. 1992;146:1297-1301

[112] Gupta N, Grover H, Bansal I, et al. Neonatal cranial sonography: Ultrasound findings in neonatal meningitis-a pictorial review. Quantitative Imaging in Medicine and Surgery. 2017;7:123-131

[113] Raju VS, Rao MN, Rao VS. Cranial sonography in pyogenic meningitis in neonates and infants. Journal of Tropical Pediatrics. 1995;41:68-73

[114] Yikilmaz A, Taylor GA. Sonographic findings in bacterial meningitis in neonates and young infants. Pediatric Radiology. 2008;38:129-137

[115] Schneider JF, Hanquinet S, Severino M, et al. MR imaging of neonatal brain infections. Magnetic Resonance Imaging Clinics of North America. 2011;19:761-775

[116] Jaremko JL, Moon AS, Kumbla S. Patterns of complications of neonatal and infant meningitis on MRI by organism: A 10 year review. European Journal of Radiology. 2011;80:821-827

[117] Brouwer MC, McIntyre P, Prasad K, et al. Corticosteroids for acute bacterial meningitis. Cochrane Database of Systematic Reviews. 2013;6:CD004405

[118] Spreer A, Gerber J, Hanssen M, et al. Dexamethasone increases hippocampal neuronal apoptosis in a rabbit model of *Escherichia coli* meningitis. Pediatric Research. 2006;60:210-215

[119] Ogunlesi TA, Odigwe CC, Oladapo OT. Adjuvant corticosteroids for reducing death in neonatal bacterial meningitis. Cochrane Database of Systematic Reviews. 2015;11:CD010435

[120] Wall EC, Ajdukiewicz KM, Bergman H, et al. Osmotic therapies added to antibiotics for acute bacterial meningitis. Cochrane Database of Systematic Reviews. 2018;2:CD008806

[121] Edwards MS, Baker CJ. Bacterial meningitis in the neonate: Neurologic complications. In: Kaplan SL, Weisman LE, Nordli DR, editors. UpToDate. Waltam, MA: UpToDate Inc. Available from: https://www.uptodate.com [Accessed: September 16, 2018]

[122] Unhanand M, Mustafa MM, McCracken GH Jr, et al. Gram-negative enteric bacillary meningitis: A twenty-one-year experience. The Journal of Pediatrics. 1993;122:15-21

[123] Kumar R, Singhi P, Dekate P, et al. Meningitis related ventriculitis— Experience from a tertiary care centre

in northern India. Indian Journal of
Pediatrics. 2015;**82**:315-320

[124] Tibussek D, Sinclair A, Yau I,
et al. Late-onset group B streptococcal
meningitis has cerebrovascular
complications. The Journal of Pediatrics.
2015;**166**:1187-1192

[125] Klinger G, Chin CN, Beyene J, et al.
Predicting the outcome of neonatal
bacterial meningitis. Pediatrics.
2000;**106**:477-482

[126] Baş AY, Demirel N, Aydin M,
et al. Pneumococcal meningitis in the
newborn period in a prevaccination
era: A 10-year experience at a tertiary
intensive care unit. The Turkish Journal
of Pediatrics. 2011;**53**:142-148

[127] Heath PT, Schuchat A. Perinatal
group B streptococcal disease. Best
Practice & Research. Clinical Obstetrics
& Gynaecology. 2007;**21**:411-424

[128] Oster G, Edelsberg J, Hennegan
K, et al. Prevention of group B
streptococcal disease in the first
3 months of life: Would routine
maternal immunization during
pregnancy be cost-effective? Vaccine.
2014;**32**:4778-4785

[129] Lassi ZS, Bhutta ZA. Community-
based intervention packages for
reducing maternal and neonatal
morbidity and mortality and improving
neonatal outcomes. Cochrane
Database of Systematic Reviews.
2015;**3**:CD007754

[130] Borghesi A, Stronati M. Strategies
for the prevention of hospital-acquired
infections in the neonatal intensive care
unit. The Journal of Hospital Infection.
2008;**68**:293-300

Chapter 4

Platelets in the Newborn

Ijeoma Esiaba, Iman Mousselli, Giulia M. Faison,
Danilyn M. Angeles and Danilo S. Boskovic

Abstract

Platelets were first described in the mid-nineteenth century. Since then, their roles were identified in hemostasis and thrombosis, inflammation, leukocyte interactions, angiogenesis, and cancer growth. But there is little information about such platelet functions in the newborn. Several studies highlighted some platelet differences between newborns and adults. Yet, in spite of these differences, healthy newborns appear to be adequately protected. A number of factors, however, were reported to negatively affect neonatal platelets. These include maternal hypertensive disorders or infections, neonatal asphyxia or respiratory distress, therapies such as ampicillin or indomethacin, and treatment modalities such as ventilators, nitric oxide, or extracorporeal membrane oxygenation (ECMO). Their effects on newborn platelets are usually transitory, lasting from several hours to a few days or weeks. If these effects are well characterized, they could serve as reporters for diagnosis and monitoring during therapy. Careful studies of neonatal platelets are needed to improve the understanding of basic physiology and pathophysiology in this cohort and to identify possible targets for intervention and therapy.

Keywords: platelet function, hemostasis, prematurity, platelet transfusion, newborn, sepsis, ECMO

1. Introduction

Platelets are small discoid cellular particles, produced by megakaryocytes, and best known for their role in thrombus or platelet plug formation. Since their initial description in the mid-nineteenth century, further details have emerged about their structure and function. More recently, their roles in processes as wide ranging as tissue repair and wound healing, angiogenesis, tumor killing, tumor growth and metastasis, inflammation, and host defense have come to light [1, 2]. Platelets perform these varied functions and diverse interactions because of several receptors and ligands on their surface, and a store of over 300 proteins within their cytoplasm and granules. With newer technological advances, more platelet functions were discovered and the mechanisms for some of them are now clearer.

Platelets mediate primary hemostasis, a dynamic process involving several reactions resulting in thrombus formation. Initially, platelets aggregate to form a platelet plug at the site of injury [3, 4]. In secondary hemostasis, thrombin is generated after a cascade of enzymatic reactions. The generated thrombin subsequently cleaves fibrinogen to fibrin [5]. Fibrin spontaneously polymerizes forming a fibrous network which stabilizes the platelet plug [6]. The process of tertiary hemostasis, or fibrinolysis, restricts clot formation to the site of injury, dissolves clots after the

damaged endothelium has been repaired, and prevents the formation of pathologic thrombi [7, 8]. These reactions are tightly regulated to minimize the risk of
either bleeding or thrombosis. Components of the hemostatic system are usually
preformed and circulate in their respective inactive forms. Apart from their role in
hemostasis, some of these factors also play a role in other physiological processes
such as embryonic development, angiogenesis, or immunity [9].

Most of the information about platelets is based on studies conducted in adults
or in animal models. Despite recognized roles of platelets in processes as wide
ranging as inflammation and angiogenesis, information about these roles of neonatal platelets is limited. However, clinical observations suggest that there likely
are some functional differences between neonatal and adult platelets. Newborns
are at greater risk of contracting infections and may not cope adequately with
inflammatory stresses [10]. New blood vessels are formed to meet the demands of
rapidly growing tissues. The roles of platelets in these processes and reactions in
the newborn are not yet well described. Additionally, certain prematurity-related
morbidities such as intraventricular hemorrhage, retinopathy of prematurity, and
necrotizing enterocolitis are associated with bleeding and inflammation [11, 12].
Platelets or their functional deficits are believed to be involved in these disorders.
Studying platelet function in the newborn is difficult, but emerging methodological
approaches requiring small volumes of newborn's blood are making such studies
feasible. Following a general description of platelet structure and functions, this
review will highlight documented differences in the newborn.

2. Platelet structure and functions

Platelets mediate primary hemostasis and play roles in procoagulant and fibrinolytic processes [13]. They are nonnucleated fragments derived from bone marrow
megakaryocytes. The adult human produces about 10^{11} platelets daily, rising by
more than 20-fold during increased need [14]. In the fetus and neonate, platelets are
produced largely in the liver and spleen [15, 16]. Thrombopoietin maintains platelet
homeostasis by regulating thrombopoiesis [17, 18]. The resting platelet is disk shaped
with a diameter of about 1.5 μm and a lifespan of 7–10 days [19]. Its surface does not
promote coagulation or aggregation. In circulation, the platelets' resting state is further supported by the release of prostacyclin and nitric oxide from endothelial cells, by
the expression of CD39 (an ADPase) on the endothelial surface, and by the inability of
normal plasma vWF to bind spontaneously to the platelet surface [20].

Platelets have a complex internal structure with a series of organelles. Lacking
a nucleus, they nevertheless contain some nucleic acid in the form of ribonucleic
acid (RNA), which is used for synthesis of new proteins, especially during or after
platelet activation [21]. The secretory granules comprise the α-granules and dense
or δ-granules. The α-granules contain adhesion molecules important for platelet
interactions with other platelets and blood cells, angiogenic and mitogenic factors,
plasma proteins, and several factors relevant for coagulation and fibrinolysis [22].
The dense- or δ-granules contain non-protein molecules such as adenosine diphos-
phate (ADP), adenosine triphosphate (ATP), calcium and serotonin [22]. These
play central roles in amplification of platelet activation and aggregation and in
modulation of vascular endothelium and leukocyte functions. Within lysosomes are
membrane proteins and acid hydrolases that digest the material in platelet aggregates through hydrolytic degradation [23]. Over 300 proteins are secreted from
these granules during activation [24]. In the unstimulated platelets, the granule
contents remain internalized. When stimulated, however, platelets release such
contents through an open canalicular system [25].

A number of factors and agonists can stimulate platelets. These include shear stress during blood flow, agonists such as thrombin, collagen, or ADP, and recognition of and interaction with viruses, bacteria, or damaged vascular endothelium [26, 27]. Typically, platelet activation is triggered when there is a break in the vascular endothelium. The activated platelets first adhere to the damaged endothelium by binding to von Willebrand factor (vWF) through its surface membrane glycoprotein Ib (GPIb). Further interactions of platelet glycoprotein VI (GPVI) with fibrillary collagen and platelet $\beta1$ integrin with laminin, collagen, and fibronectin maintain platelet adhesion to exposed extracellular matrix [8].

Following activation, platelet membrane phospholipid distribution changes to include exposure of phosphatidylserine on the outer surface, thus promoting the condensation of vitamin K-dependent coagulation factors on this surface, and inducing the activation of the procoagulant cascade [28]. Additionally, a rearrangement of the cytoskeleton leads to a change in platelet structure [29] from the resting discoid form, via an intermediate spherical shape, to a fully activated amoeboid form with numerous extending pseudopodia able to interact with some nearby surfaces [29]. Meanwhile, the contents of α- and δ-granules are released into the immediate environment, further amplifying the original activation signal [23]. As a result, in response to a number of biological mediators, the activated platelets adhere to each other, to leukocytes and endothelial cells, and to components of the sub-endothelial matrix [30].

During extension of platelet plug formation, activated platelets accumulate on top of the initial monolayer of platelets bound to collagen of the sub-endothelium [3]. Expressed receptors on each platelet allow binding of agonists such as ADP, thrombin, and thromboxane A_2, which are released from activated platelets [31]. Consequently, more platelets are recruited to the site of injury, thereby consolidating the initial hemostatic plug. Binding of fibrin to aggregated platelets through activated receptor glycoprotein GPIIb/IIIa (integrin $\alpha_{IIb}\beta_3$) helps to further stabilize the hemostatic plug [32].

Several proteins are released during platelet aggregation at a damaged blood vessel surface [22]. Some are believed to be responsible for repair of damaged blood vessels and development of new ones. Although precise mechanisms are not well understood, it was suggested that platelets are necessary for formation of new blood vessels [33]. Supporting this are observations of reduced retinal neovascularization in a mouse hypoxia-induced retinal angiogenesis model due to thrombocytopenia or in response to treatment with inhibitors of platelet aggregation [33]. In this context, platelet granules are believed to contain pro- and anti-angiogenic compounds [34, 35]. Similarly, platelet interactions with cancer cells appear to play a role in the development of metastases and tumor angiogenesis [36]. While cerebrovascular remodeling is known to occur in the newborn in the first few postnatal weeks [37], the roles of platelets in this developmental process are not yet well described.

Platelets may also play a role in newborn's inflammatory processes and host defense. Neonates are generally believed to be at least partially immunologically incompetent and susceptible to a variety of infections. In this context, it is of interest that platelets have toll-like receptors (TLRs) that directly recognize and interact with a number of microorganisms or their products. Platelets may be responsible for killing microbes directly by phagocytosis, by release of microbicidal agents, or as sentinels communicating information about microbial encounters to cells of the innate immune system [15]. Bacterial infections, found in preterm newborns admitted to the neonatal intensive care unit (NICU), appear similar to infections found in adults with severe neutropenia [38]. This suggests reduced neutrophil functions in these babies. Neonates rely heavily on innate immunity for protection because their adaptive immunity is not yet fully developed [39]. Neutrophils are usually the first cells to be recruited to infection sites. They kill pathogens by various mechanisms including (a) direct phagocytosis and chemical killing by degranulation and (b) by formation of neutrophil extracellular traps (NETs) [40]. Recent studies showed that platelet interactions with neutrophils are important for optimal neutrophil functions [41–44]. One such aspect of neutrophil function involves their chemotaxis and extravasation to sites of infection. Platelets were observed to act as "pathfinders" guiding neutrophils to infection sites, and platelet inhibition resulted in poor neutrophil chemotaxis [45, 46]. Interaction of platelets with leukocytes may induce inflammation. Understanding the role and mechanisms involved in platelet-leukocyte interactions in the newborn, particularly those born prematurely, could lead to development of more rational approaches to morbidities common to this group.

3. Newborn platelets

Thrombopoietin, a protein regulator of platelet synthesis and homeostasis [18], was detected in the fetal liver as early as the sixth week of gestation [18]. In turn, megakaryocytes, the precursor cells that form and release platelets into circulation, were detected in the liver and circulation at the eighth week [19]. The megakaryocyte numbers were observed to be, at least in part, inversely correlated to gestational age, so that healthy preterm newborns characteristically have higher levels, while levels in healthy full term newborns and adults are similar [47, 48]. Neonatal megakaryocyte progenitor cells are more sensitive and have higher proliferative potential in response to thrombopoietin compared to adult cells, and this sensitivity is even greater in preterm newborns [49]. However, neonatal megakaryocytes, tending to be smaller and with a lower ploidy than adult cells, produce fewer platelets per megakaryocyte [48, 50, 51]. Newborn and adult platelets are ultra-structurally similar [52, 53] and contain comparable membrane receptor glycoproteins (GPs) [54] and thromboxane receptors [55]. However, newborn platelets tend to include more immature forms, with the ability to form fewer pseudopods, fewer developed microtubular structures, and fewer α-granules [53]. Additionally, neonatal platelets have fewer adrenergic receptors [56]. Although they store comparably adult levels of ADP, ATP and serotonin in their dense granules, the overall dense granule release during platelet activation is lower in the newborn [57].

Platelet count is dependent on gestational age, increasing during fetal life, but usually reaches the expected adult range of 150,000 to 450,000/μL [58] from about 22 weeks of gestation [59]. The percentage of reticulated platelets, an indication of newly produced platelets, is higher in the newborn circulation [60], while the mean platelet volume (MPV), a measure of platelet size, tends to be comparable to adults.

Platelet adhesion to, and coverage of, sub-endothelial extracellular matrix is higher in the newborns than in adults [61, 62]. This is in spite of comparable collagen binding or platelet aggregation [61]. The enhanced neonatal platelet adhesion is believed to be mediated by the neonatal plasma von Willebrand factor (vWF) [61], which was reported to include unusually large multimers [63, 64]. Nevertheless, compared to full-term newborns, platelet adhesion tended to be lower in earlier gestational age neonates [62]. In part, these observations could help to explain how hemostatic function is usually maintained in full-term newborns, despite decreased intrinsic platelet activation, and why the preterm neonates are progressively decompensated the earlier their gestational age.

The phospholipid content and baseline exposure of platelet surface phosphatidylserine is comparable in adults and newborns [65, 66]. However, more platelet microparticles are generated and more phosphatidylserine molecules are exposed in the term and preterm platelets when thrombin or calcium ionophores were used as activators [67]. Microparticles or exposed phosphatidylserine is expected to induce a procoagulant state. Yet, the procoagulant activity, especially in the preterm newborn, is generally lower despite the higher levels of generated microparticles and exposed phosphatidylserine [67]. Supplementing neonatal plasma with coagulation factors improves its procoagulant activity so that it becomes comparable to adults. This implies that newborn platelets can often present adequate procoagulant surface, but the apparent poor activity may in part be due to a deficiency of humoral factors [68].

P-selectin expression, as an index of α-granule secretion, was reported lower in newborn platelets compared to adults, especially in the <30 week gestation group [69, 70]. Neonatal dense granule secretion, measured by secreted serotonin, was similar to that in adults when inositol triphosphate, 1-oleoyl-2-acetyl-glycerol, or thrombin was used as an agonist. Collagen-mediated stimulation, however, resulted in lower serotonin secretion in cord blood, although the number of dense granules in adults and neonates was found to be similar [57, 68]. GPIIb/IIIa receptors are expressed early during gestation. Yet, the fraction of active GPIIb/IIIa in neonatal cord and peripheral blood is lower compared to adults [69].

During the first few days of life, platelet activation appears to be less effective, as indicated by flow cytometric studies [69]. However, these activation profiles approach the adult patterns between the tenth and the fourteenth day of life [71]. Proposed explanations for this observed hypo-responsiveness include: relative deficiencies of phospholipid metabolism including thromboxane production, differential regulation of GPIIb/IIIa activation, impaired mobilization of calcium and intracellular signaling, impaired granule secretion, and lower aggregation [72]. These could result from lower intrinsic signal transduction in neonatal platelets [72]. Such effects are further enhanced by lower expression of protease-activated receptor-1 (PAR-1) and PAR-4 [73, 74], which mediate thrombin-dependent platelet activation.

Various components of the hemostatic system in the fetus and neonate are qualitatively and quantitatively different from those in adults [8]. Such differences could be explained either by lower synthesis, higher clearance, or higher consumption [75, 76]. Although the hemostatic system is sometimes thought to be incomplete at birth [72], it nevertheless appears to be adequate for the majority of healthy full-term newborns.

4. Perinatal factors affecting platelet function in the newborn

Acquired platelet dysfunctions are common during the neonatal period especially in preterm newborns. These disorders are usually secondary to perinatal or neonatal conditions such as maternal and neonatal state of health, presence of infections, medications given to mother or to newborn, or interventions for the newborn (**Tables 1** and **2**). Platelet count and function are usually restored several hours or days after the triggering condition is removed.

4.1 Prenatal and maternal factors associated with neonatal platelet dysfunction

There are several maternal factors that can impact neonatal platelet function especially during the days preceding delivery. These include maternal hypertensive disorders and prenatal use of aspirin, magnesium sulfate, or antibiotics.

Hypertensive disorders of pregnancy are associated with platelet dysfunctions in the newborn. Pregnancy-induced hypertension (PIH) is a risk factor for early onset thrombocytopenia in the newborn [77]. This is especially true for babies born prior to 36 weeks of gestation [78, 79]. Neonatal platelet counts tend to be inversely correlated to maternal blood pressure [79]. These platelets also exhibited lower adhesion properties [80]. Babies with low birth weight, meconium aspiration, or infections are also at greater risk for thrombocytopenia [81, 82]. Flow cytometric analyses of platelets from premature newborns from preeclamptic mothers demonstrated lower expression of

Factor	Effect on newborn platelet
Hypertension in mother	• Reduced platelet adhesion and surface coverage [80]
	• Low platelet count [78, 79]
	• Decreased secretion and expression of CD62P, CD63, and CD36 [83]
	• Increased expression of CD62P and CD63 [84]
	• Low platelet and megakaryocyte counts [84]
Magnesium sulfate (prenatal)	• Reduced ADP-mediated platelet aggregation [97]
Low dose aspirin (prenatal)	• Reduced platelet aggregation [95]
	• No change in platelet count and aggregation [92, 93]
	• Reduced thromboxane B2 production [94]
Indomethacin	• Prolonged bleeding time and gastrointestinal hemorrhage [104, 105]
	• Reduced prostacyclin and prostaglandin levels [104]
	• Abnormal platelet aggregation up to 4 days after medication [106]
Ibuprofen	• Prolonged PFA-100 closure time [108]

Table 1.
Maternal factors affecting platelets in the newborn.

Neonatal factor	Effect on newborn platelet
Nitric oxide	• Abnormal thromboelastogram values [109]
	• Prolonged prothrombin time [109]
	• Prolonged bleeding time [111]
Therapeutic hypothermia	• Abnormal thromboelastogram values, associated with bleeding [199]
	• Reduced platelet count [123, 200]
	• Prolonged bleeding time and PFA 100 closure time [201]
Asphyxia and RDS	• Reduced platelet count [113, 118, 120]
	• High MPV and PDW [113, 117]
	• Increased thrombopoietin level [118]
	• Increased thromboxane level [120]
Mechanical ventilation	• Reduced platelet count [121]
Extracorporeal membrane oxygenation (ECMO)	• Reduced platelet count [125, 126]
	• Reduced platelet activation [126]

RDS, respiratory distress syndrome; MPV, mean platelet volume; PDW, platelet distribution width.

Table 2.
Neonatal factors affecting platelets in the newborn.

CD62P (P-selectin), CD63 (platelet activation marker), or CD36 (platelet glycoprotein IV (GPIV)) after thrombin stimulation, compared to full-term neonates [83]. However, when compared to other similar preterms, the expression of platelet CD62P and CD63 was relatively higher in newborns from preeclamptic mothers [84]. Additionally, this cohort was also characterized by lower platelet and megakaryocyte counts [84], implying possible disturbances in platelet production [85]. Infants born to hypertensive mothers tend to be hypoxic [86]. Animal model studies suggest that hypoxia tends to favor erythropoiesis over megakaryopoiesis, leading to lower platelet counts [87].

Low dose aspirin (LDA), about 60–100 mg, is sometimes given to pregnant women, who are at risk of developing a hypertensive disorder, or whose fetus has intrauterine growth restriction [88, 89]. Aspirin inhibits cyclooxygenase, which catalyzes the initial steps in conversion of arachidonic acid to prostaglandins and thromboxanes [90]. Thromboxane A2 (TxA2) serves to amplify the signal during platelet activation [91]. Nevertheless, while some reports suggest that prenatal aspirin does not alter cord blood platelet count and aggregation [92] or thromboxane B2 (TxB2) inhibition [93], others challenge this with clear TxB2 differences in newborns of mothers exposed to LDA even several days after the medication was stopped [94]. This apparent contradiction may be resolved by taking into account the actual timing of LDA treatment prior to delivery. It was noted that newborn platelet dysfunction, including reduced collagen-stimulated platelet aggregation, is generally observable if the mother had aspirin within a week of delivery [95]. In this context, aspirin also increases the risk for mucocutaneous bleeding in the newborn, especially if the mother took it within five days of delivery [72, 95].

While aspirin is perhaps the best described with respect to its potential to alter platelet functions, it is not the only drug to do so. Indomethacin, given to the mother as a tocolytic, increased the risk of subsequent neonatal intraventricular hemorrhage (IVH) [96], presumably by affecting cerebral blood flow and by altering platelet and neutrophil functions. Similarly, platelets in newborns, from mothers receiving tocolytic magnesium sulfate, tended to be less effective in forming aggregates in response to ADP-mediated activation, but not so in response to collagen stimulation [97].

4.2 Postnatal and neonatal factors associated with platelet dysfunction in the newborn

Neonatal infections tend to lead to platelet consumption. This is implied by the observed upregulation of thrombopoietin and elevated megakaryocyte progenitor cells in septic newborns [98]. Reduced platelet adhesion was also reported in such neonates [99]. However, enhanced granule secretion and aggregate formation in response to agonists during experimental conditions [100] suggest that these circulating platelets may already be to some extent primed and not in their resting state. Furthermore, neonates born following chorioamnionitis had significantly higher levels of soluble P-selectin and higher CD40L (CD40 ligand, able to bind CD40 protein on antigen presenting cells) on their platelets [101].

Antibiotics are often used to treat infections and sepsis, and some of them could alter hemostatic responses. Prolonged template bleeding and PFA-100 closure times were correlated with duration and dosage of neonatal ampicillin treatment [102, 103].

Nonsteroidal anti-inflammatory drugs (NSAIDs) are known to affect platelet function in adults. Yet, they are sometimes given to newborns as a treatment for patent ductus arteriosus (PDA). Indomethacin is associated with prolonged bleeding time and gastrointestinal bleeding in preterm newborns [104]. These effects tend to last up to 48 h [105], but normal platelet values are restored about the tenth day [106]. Nevertheless, in preterm newborns with intracranial hemorrhage, indomethacin administration for treatment of PDA did not extend the hemorrhage [107]. In contrast, ibuprofen treatment is associated with prolonged PFA-100 closure time, but not with altered bleeding time [108].

Inhaled nitric oxide (NO) is used as a selective pulmonary vasodilator to treat hypoxemic respiratory failure or pulmonary hypertension in newborns ($\geq$34 week gestation) [109]. Inhaled NO prolongs bleeding time in adults [110]. Persistent pulmonary hypertension and treatment with inhaled NO were reported to alter neonatal platelet thromboelastogram (TEG) values [109]. Bleeding time was also prolonged in such babies [111]. These clinical tests, however, returned to normal after about 24 h of stopping therapy. It is of interest that newborns receiving NO therapy did not experience increased risk of intracranial hemorrhage [72]. Nitric oxide is known to inhibit platelet adhesion and aggregation by inhibiting GPIIb/IIIa activation [110]. A reduction in expressed P-selectin and activated GPIIb/IIIa on collagen-stimulated platelets was reported after NO treatment in adults and newborns [112].

Term newborns who were small for gestational age tended to have lower platelet counts but higher mean platelet volumes (MPVs) [113, 114]. A similar pattern was also observed in asphyxiated term newborns [113]. MPV is a measure of average platelet size [115] and may serve as a marker of platelet production, consumption, or severity of some disorder of bone marrow, thrombosis, or infection [116, 117]. For example, MPV was elevated in preterm newborns with respiratory distress [117], suggesting potential issues in platelet production, consumption, or both. Asphyxia is associated with upregulation of thrombopoietin concentration, which in turn is negatively correlated to platelet count up to the 7th day of life [118]. Thrombocytopenia, however, when associated with perinatal asphyxia, does not tend to resolve until about the 19th to 21st day of life [119]. Increased thromboxane levels in asphyxiated newborns [120] suggest platelet activation, and possibly consumption, as an explanation for the observed thrombocytopenia. Hypoxia leads to preferential upregulation of erythropoiesis over megakaryopoiesis [87, 114], consistent with elevated thrombopoietin observed [118].

Mechanical ventilation is generally used to resuscitate hypoxic or asphyxiated newborns. It was reported that mechanical ventilation led to reduced platelet counts in newborns with respiratory distress, or in rabbit models, regardless of the oxygen concentration used [121]. However, using newborn piglet models of hypoxia, it was found that various platelet indices were affected particularly by high oxygen level used [122]. Resuscitation with 100% oxygen led to enhanced collagen-stimulated platelet aggregation, while using 18–21% oxygen did not do so [122].

To prevent permanent brain damage following perinatal asphyxia, the newborns are sometimes treated with therapeutic hypothermia. The hypothermia treatment, in turn, led to decreased platelet counts, but had an overall protective effect by reducing risk of cerebral hemorrhage [123] and restoring other hemostatic parameters [124]. Similarly, extracorporeal membrane oxygenation (ECMO) is used to rescue term newborns with persistent pulmonary hypertension, asphyxia, or congenital diaphragmatic hernia [125]. Platelet counts and rates of activation were reduced during ECMO therapy, and were not fully restored with transfusion, until several hours post-ECMO [125, 126].

5. Platelets and sepsis

Sepsis is a complex syndrome characterized by disordered immune, endocrine, and metabolic responses to infection [127]. The exaggerated responses can lead to multi-organ failure (MOF), shock, and death [127]. Sepsis is generally considered if a documented or suspected infection is present with at least one additional finding (e.g., fever/hypothermia, elevated heart rate, and leukocytosis/leukopenia). In contrast to infection, however, sepsis is defined by additional evidence of organ dysfunction and a dysregulated host immune response [127], its key features. Notably, interactions between the innate immune system and the hemostatic system, including platelets and coagulation factors, were identified as principal steps in the pathogenesis of sepsis. Progressive thrombocytopenia and coagulopathy are strong negative prognostic findings in severe sepsis and have recently been included in the updated definition of the disease [127]. Platelets are able to release cytokines, recruit leukocytes, interact with bacteria and the endothelium, and contribute to formation of microthrombi [128]. These processes are adaptive and protective in the context of

Biomarker	Association	References
Thrombocytopenia	Mortality	[133]
Impaired platelet function	MOF, mortality	[132, 133]
Impaired platelet aggregation	ALI	[133]
P-selectin	MOF	[133]
Platelet-neutrophil aggregates	Sepsis progression	[132, 133]
Immature platelet fraction	MOF	[133]
MOF, multi-organ failure; ALI, acute lung injury; TPO, thrombopoietin.		

Table 3.
Platelet-related biomarkers of sepsis severity in human studies.

a localized infection, but may become dysregulated and "maladaptive" during sepsis, contributing to organ damage [129]. A low platelet count is a well-known biomarker for disease severity. More recently, attention has been focused on the active role of platelets in the pathogenesis of multi-organ failure.

The correlation between thrombocytopenia and sepsis is well documented [130]. Platelet count below <50,000/μL is a strong negative prognostic marker in patients with sepsis and is thought to result from platelet activation and consumption [131, 132]. A number of platelet function markers were proposed as biomarkers for sepsis correlating with its severity [133] (**Table 3**).

Moreover, platelets interact with neutrophils in the formation of NETs (neutrophil extracellular traps) resulting in the trapping and killing of pathogens [133]. They also play a central role in driving and modulating host inflammatory and immune responses, influencing directly the function of endothelial cells, neutrophils, and lymphocytes [134]. Platelets are the most numerous blood cells with immune function, able to interact with bacteria in several ways: (1) direct interaction between platelet glycoproteins and bacterial surface proteins, as occurs between GPIb and *S. sanguis* SrpA [134]; (2) indirect interactions, such as the interaction of platelet $\alpha_{IIb}\beta_3$ with fibrinogen to which the clumping factors of *S. aureus* bind [134]; and (3) upon activation, platelets release a series of factors which can modulate the immune response or have direct microbicidal effects. For example, released thrombin-induced platelet microbicidal protein (tPMP-1) can directly lyse bacteria, like *S. aureus* [134].

5.1 Conclusions

In addition to hemostasis, platelets actively participate in the innate immune defense system. Participating in the recognition of pathogens, signal transduction, or the release of cytokines/chemokines, they reveal a functional similarity with leucocytes in sepsis and septic shock. There is abundant evidence that platelets can influence key host responses to sepsis. Further studies are needed to address the effects of platelet transfusion or inhibition toward sepsis prevention and treatment particularly in the newborn.

6. Platelets in neonates with extracorporeal membrane oxygenation

Extracorporeal membrane oxygenators are used to provide gas exchange in severe respiratory failure employing venovenous (VV) circuits or, increasingly, if associated with concurrent cardiac failure, veno-arterial (VA) circuits, while waiting for organ recovery to occur. Support by cardiopulmonary bypass (CPB) systems decreased the morbidity and mortality of children, especially those who require surgery for life-threatening anatomical heart defects [135, 136]. ECMO contributed to decreased mortality for children with severe cardiac or respiratory failure [137, 138]. While annually thousands of neonates are helped by ECMO support, thromboembolic complications also frequently occur [139]. Nevertheless, for many neonatal patients, survival is made possible only because of ECMO support [136]. ECMO is used to treat a variety of conditions in neonatal patients, including respiratory and cardiac failure as a result of persistent pulmonary hypertension (PPHN), congenital diaphragmatic hernia (CDH), meconium aspiration syndrome (MAS), respiratory distress syndrome (RDS), pneumonia, severe air-leak syndromes, or sepsis [140].

Both bleeding and clotting complications can occur during ECMO support, often coexist in the same patient, and are associated with significant morbidity and mortality [141]. Moreover, patients requiring ECMO are critically ill, thus making it difficult to distinguish the relative contributions of the underlying pathology from that of the ECMO circuit as such. Rates of reported ECMO-associated venous thromboembolism (VTE) in general population, ranging from 18 to 85% in various centers, may be at least partly dependent on anticoagulation regimens [141]. Severe hemorrhage is reported in nearly 40% and intracranial hemorrhage in 16–21% of patients [142, 143]. At the same time, there is broad variation in practice, without clear consensus, on the administration and monitoring of anticoagulation during ECMO, or the management of ECMO-related hemorrhage and VTE [144].

Activation of the coagulation system is initiated by the exposure of blood to foreign synthetic surfaces and by shear stresses of the circuit, especially from device pumps. The shift to a pro-coagulant state appears to be mediated primarily by thrombin, while an excessive fibrinolytic tendency is mediated by plasmin, resulting in a consumption of clotting factors, impaired platelet function, thrombocytopenia, and fibrinolysis [145]. Initial fibrinogen deposition and subsequent activation of coagulation and complement factors allow platelets and leukocytes to adhere to oxygenator surfaces further enhancing thrombin generation. Such changes contribute to higher rates of thrombosis in these patients [145]. Meanwhile, several of a series of processes contribute to higher bleeding rates. (a) Primary hemostasis is impaired because of platelet dysfunction and loss of key adhesive molecules. (b) Shear stress causes the development of an acquired von Willebrand defect. (c) Widespread fibrin deposits on surfaces trigger an enhanced fibrinolytic response. (d) Administration of systemic anticoagulation, required to maintain circuit patency, raises bleeding risks [146].

Balancing the relative risks of bleeding and thrombosis can be difficult. Factors related to patient's illness, the extracorporeal support, and the interplay between pro-inflammatory and anti-inflammatory processes vary among patients.

6.1 Platelet dysfunction during ECMO

If the ECMO circuit is primed only with crystalloid or RBCs and plasma, then dilutional coagulopathy and dilutional thrombocytopenia develop as the ECMO is initiated. Dilutional coagulopathy is generally not severe, but will complement the systemic anticoagulation. Dilutional thrombocytopenia, however, may further aggravate any preexisting thrombocytopenia or platelet dysfunction, frequently present in premature neonates. Accurate assessment of platelet function under these circumstances can be difficult, further complicating evaluation of patient's bleeding or thrombotic potential. Impairment of platelets can occur as early as 15 min after starting ECMO and last until it is discontinued [125].

Platelets adhere to the protein-coated monolayer of the ECMO circuit surfaces and interact with activated components of the coagulation and complement systems [147]. Elevated shear flow from the ECMO circuit causes some platelet receptor shedding. Of particular interest are the losses of key platelet adhesion glycoproteins GPI and GPVI, and the associated reduction of high molecular weight vWF multimers. GPI serves as a receptor for vWF and GPVI as a receptor for collagen [126]. Adhesive proteins, vWF, and fibrinogen assist platelets to bind to damaged vessel wall surface and to other platelets [148]. As platelet thrombus is being formed, the prothrombinase enzyme complex assembles on the activated platelet surfaces to produce thrombin. In turn, thrombin cleaves fibrinogen to form fibrin, which spontaneously polymerizes to form the fibrin meshwork, which further strengthens the thrombus [149]. Consequently, shedding of GPI and loss of high molecular weight vWF lead to dysfunctional platelet responses to vascular injury. This persists despite platelet transfusion and throughout the period of ECMO use [126]. Subsequently, lower levels of platelet aggregation are observed by light aggregometry using various agonists including ADP, ristocetin, collagen, or epinephrine [150]. Such decreased potential for platelet aggregation may lead to increased bleeding risk particularly when combined with the effects of anticoagulants or antiplatelet agents. Flow cytometry of blood, from those receiving ECMO support, showed severely reduced membrane-bound P-selectin (CD62P) and CD63, both of which modulate platelet spreading [151].

Despite reduced aggregation and lower expression of key platelet adhesion and structural molecules, there is a time-dependent platelet activation marked by increased levels of circulating matrix metalloproteinase-2 (MMP-2) and soluble P-selectin [126]. This is not associated with significant activation of the endothelium [126], but may be due to the release of platelet granules [152]. Furthermore, this time-dependent platelet activation is also accompanied by platelet receptor shedding and the release of platelet microparticles (PMPs) [153]. These are small cell-derived particles, typically 0.1–1 μm in size, that are produced from activated platelets in situations of shear stress [154]. While these PMPs can present a prothrombotic surface, it is not clear whether they are a major contributor to the prothrombotic phenotype or to the pathogenesis of ECMO-associated coagulopathy [153].

6.2 Platelet counts during ECMO

Thrombocytopenia is common in critically ill patients. A constant shear force, caused by the ECMO pump, is implicated in acquired platelet dysfunctions. Appropriate anticoagulation is difficult to achieve during ECMO since severe thrombocytopenia of <50,000/μL may be present even prior to ECMO. This situation increases the practice of platelet transfusions [155]. Minimal target platelet counts vary from 25,000 to 100,000/μL between hospitals. However, if bleeding occurs or is expected, then target platelet counts are increased to 150,000/μL or higher, particularly if platelet dysfunction is suspected. As in any setting of thrombocytopenia, it is important to try and identify the cause and treat appropriately [156, 157]. Bleeding in critically ill patients with a platelet count of 30,000/μL is believed to be associated with additional disturbances of hemostasis [158]. Platelet transfusion is recommended in bleeding patients with either primary or secondary platelet abnormalities regardless of platelet counts [158]. Required thresholds for prophylactic platelet transfusions, however, are generally at platelet levels above 20,000/μL, given the requirements of invasive procedures and potential bleeding risk [158]. Many centers describe targeting a platelet count of >100,000/μL during an ECMO [159]. Research to support this practice, however, is lacking and urgently needed.

6.3 Anticoagulation during ECMO

Unfractionated heparin is the most widely used anticoagulant during ECMO [160]. Heparin levels tend to be monitored primarily indirectly by activated clotting time (ACT) [159]. While there are a number of devices that promise to describe certain characteristics of platelet function, it is not yet clear to what extent the data produced by them actually reflect the physiological platelet interactions and roles. Viscoelastic tests using rotational thromboelastometry (ROTEM) assess whole blood coagulation, and thus provide information on the dynamics of clot development, stabilization, and dissolution. Several reports suggest that ROTEM-guided coagulation management could reduce bleeding episodes in ECMO patients [160, 161]. Similarly, whole blood platelet aggregometry using the Multiplate (Roche Diagnostics, Munich, Germany) demonstrated decreased platelet aggregation in ECMO patients [161].

Other intravenous anticoagulants, such as bivalirudin and argatroban, are used increasingly, particularly if heparin-induced thrombocytopenia (HIT), heparin resistance, or allergy is suspected [162, 163]. At present, there is no clear consensus on administration and monitoring of anticoagulation during ECMO or on management of ECMO-related hemorrhage and VTE [164]. The current aim of anticoagulation is to reduce thrombin generation. This, however, increases the risk of hemorrhage. The ideal therapeutic agent, which would reduce thrombotic risk without increasing the risk of bleeding, remains elusive.

6.4 Heparin-induced thrombocytopenia

Heparin-induced thrombocytopenia (HIT) is an immune-mediated coagulation side effect of heparin therapy characterized by a prothrombotic state mediated by platelets, leukocytes, and antibodies against complexes of platelet factor 4 (PF4) with long chain heparins [165]. Rapid platelet consumption leads to thrombocytopenia. HIT was considered to be very rare in the pediatric population. However, more recent reports indicate that it occurs in children receiving unfractionated heparin therapy with an incidence similar to that seen in adults [166]. The highest incidence of pediatric HIT was found in pediatric intensive care units supporting patients following cardiac surgery [167].

At least 70 cases of reported HIT were documented in pediatric patients [168], with the majority occurring during care following cardiac surgery. HIT in children was reported to occur in all age groups, but with a bimodal distribution. The higher incidences occur a) early in life, between 0–2, and b) during puberty, between 11–17 years of age [168, 169]. The balance between the risk of procoagulant and thromboembolic events on one hand and the risk of severe, sometimes fatal, bleeding on the other hand can be very challenging in ECMO patients with HIT. Pollak et al. reported a case of HIT with evidence of small vessel arterial thrombosis in a 5-day-old newborn receiving ECMO for congenital diaphragmatic hernia. It was assumed that the leading cause of death in this patient was massive disseminated intravascular coagulation. In this case, however, it is more likely that repeated platelet transfusions proved fatal and, retrospectively speaking, should have been avoided [170]. Although HIT is a recognizable and treatable complication, its relative infrequency increases the risk for delayed diagnosis leading to significant morbidity.

Diagnostic studies for HIT tend to be unreliable. Therefore, early intervention using alternative anticoagulants is a crucial step when HIT is suspected. This can hopefully lead to improved outcomes in these patients. Treatment of confirmed or suspected HIT in patients on ECMO includes removing unfractionated heparin, and possibly the entire ECMO circuit. Certain modern ECMO circuit components are heparin bonded in an effort to reduce immune reactivity to foreign surfaces [171–173]. If platelet recovery does not occur after withdrawal of heparin, it is possible that ongoing exposure to heparin bonding may be a factor [173]. Options for alternative anticoagulation if HIT is suspected include direct thrombin inhibitors (argatroban and bivalirudin) as well as short heparinoids (fondaparinux and danaparoid) [162, 174].

6.5 Conclusions

The predominant challenge for the clinician caring for a patient on ECMO is making an informed assessment of bleeding and clotting risks. The goal is to minimize bleeding and transfusion requirements while avoiding formation of micro or macro thrombi either in the circuit or within the patient's cardiovascular system [175]. Assessment of the patient's hemostasis includes consideration of the pathophysiology, type and severity of organ failure, and extent of tissue trauma during cannulation. A holistic approach to hemostatic management is needed to balance all these factors. ROTEM and whole blood platelet aggregometry provide rapid information on whole blood coagulation, and may be helpful in providing blood product support, factor replacement, anti-coagulation therapy and anti-fibrinolytics. Further research using ROTEM and whole blood platelet aggregometry in ECMO patients is needed to demonstrate efficacy in support of real-time hemostatic management in this cohort.

7. Platelet transfusions in neonates

Transfusion of blood products in neonates is not an uncommon practice in neonatal intensive care units. Extremely premature neonates (<28 week gestation) or extremely low birth weight (ELBW) infants (<1000 g) receive at least one packed red blood cell (pRBC) transfusion per hospital admission [176]. Platelet transfusions are also quite prevalent in ELBW infants, occurring in up to 90% of those weighing less than 750 g [177]. Unfortunately, while platelet transfusions for thrombocytopenia may be helpful, they are not without risk. Further, because the guidelines for transfusion thresholds in neonates are not based on a well-developed body of evidence, there is considerable variability in circumstances for such transfusions, and in particular clinical scenarios triggering them.

Thrombocytopenia is defined by a platelet count of less than 150,000/μL, and is further sub-classified as mild (100,000–149,000/μL), moderate (50,000–99,000/μL), or severe (<50,000/μL) [178]. The reference values for very low birth weight (VLBW) babies (<1500 g), however, remain controversial [179]. Thrombocytopenia affects 18–35% of all neonates in the neonatal intensive care unit [180, 181] and up to 73% of ELBW infants [182]. While clinical significance of platelet counts between 100,000 and 150,000/μL is debatable, it is well known that platelet counts below 20,000/μL are associated with increased risk of hemorrhage, at least in the adult population [183]. The relationship between thrombocytopenia and hemorrhage, however, remains one of the associations. It is not clear that neonatal thrombocytopenia directly causes hemorrhagic events [184].

Thrombocytopenia may be described by time of onset, where early onset (occurring in the first 72 h of life) is distinguished from late onset (occurring after the first 72 h of life) [179, 184]. In the premature population, the early onset thrombocytopenia is most often mild to moderate, develops gradually, and tends to be related to causes of chronic fetal hypoxia, as seen with intra-uterine growth restriction (IUGR), pregnancy-induced hypertension (PIH), hemolysis, elevated liver enzymes and low platelet count (HELLP) syndrome, or preeclampsia [185]. In term neonates, however, platelet destruction tends to be antibody-mediated [184]. In contrast to early onset, late onset thrombocytopenia tends to be more severe, more acute, and most frequently associated with infections (NEC, sepsis, and viral infections) [184].

7.1 Indications for platelet transfusion

Due to limited understanding of neonatal platelet functions, transfusion practice in the newborn is generally extrapolated from what is recognized as beneficial within the pediatric and adult populations. However, neonates are vulnerable to particular illnesses with varying underlying disease processes. Moreover, they tend to have developmental differences in regulation of primary hemostasis [178]. Nevertheless, platelet transfusions are typically given in two distinct clinical scenarios: (a) acutely, as a life-saving procedure and (b) prophylactically, under the presumption that they diminish the risk for hemorrhage. Surprisingly, an overwhelming majority of neonatal transfusions are done prophylactically, accounting for 98% of platelet transfusions [59]. Yet, it is not clear that this practice is beneficial. Prophylactic platelet transfusion in clinically stable neonates with no active bleeding remains controversial at best [186], consistent with the wide range of national and international clinical practices by neonatologists [177]. In this context, the severity of thrombocytopenia does not correlate with increased risk of intraventricular hemorrhage (IVH), and platelet transfusion for mild to moderate thrombocytopenia does not appear to prevent or reduce the incidence of intracranial hemorrhage [183, 187].

Although adequate quantities of platelets are necessary for hemostasis, increased risk of hemorrhage appears to be dependent on factors other than thrombocytopenia alone. Additional relevant platelet parameters include functional competency, immature platelet fraction, and developmental differences in neonatal thrombopoiesis [49, 188, 189]. Underlying clinical conditions associated with increased risk of hemorrhage include: preterm premature rupture of membranes, low birth weight, sepsis, shock, pulmonary hypertension, respiratory distress, NEC, and premature gestational age [182, 190–192]. Thus, recommendations to transfuse platelets should not be solely based on thrombocytopenia, but also on the presence of such other contributory factors [178, 190]. In spite of such considerations, it appears that management of thrombocytopenia in the newborn still lacks adequately rigorous scientific basis [179].

7.2 Clinical guidelines for platelet transfusion in neonates

In the United States, there are currently no national guidelines for neonatal platelet transfusion and only two published randomized controlled trials assessing prophylactic transfusions [183, 193]. Most countries recommend therapeutic transfusion in actively bleeding neonates when platelets fall below 50,000/μL. However, there is no agreement regarding prophylactic transfusions when platelets are anywhere between 20,000 and 90,000/μL [184, 194, 195]. A wide range of thrombocytopenia thresholds are employed, tending to be markedly higher in the United States, between 50,000 and 149,000/μL [187, 196, 197]. Nonetheless, such trends are based on clinical experience and judgment, rather than on reliable and consistent data.

7.3 Adverse outcomes of platelet transfusions

A growing number of adverse effects of platelet transfusions are being documented, including but not limited to increased risk of infection, transfusion-related injuries in various organs, alloimmunization, hemolytic reactions, febrile reactions, allergic reactions, anaphylaxis, and NEC [177, 185]. Randomized controlled trials comparing thresholds for platelet transfusion in thrombocytopenic neonates concluded that the frequency of IVH is not reduced by more aggressive thresholds [183]. Additionally, platelet transfusions, themselves, are implicated in increased mortality, linking the number of transfusions with death rate [198]. This was further supported by a recent large, multicenter, randomized clinical trial suggesting that significant hemorrhage and death could be prevented by lowering thrombocytopenia transfusion thresholds from 50,000 to 25,000/μL [193].

8. Conclusions

Platelets are best known for their role in hemostasis. But beyond forming a platelet plug, they are also important in several processes such as recognition and elimination of invading microorganisms, inflammation and interaction with leukocytes, wound healing and tissue repair, angiogenesis, and even tumor growth. These are emerging areas of investigation and there is little to no information on the roles of platelets in such processes in the newborn. Although current understanding suggests that newborn platelets may be somewhat different from adult platelets, they nonetheless protect the healthy newborn adequately. Certain perinatal factors were identified to affect platelet counts and function, but the platelet dysfunctions induced by them are acquired and transitory in nature. Premature neonates are likely at greatest risk for reduced platelet counts and functions, and by extension, at greatest risk of hemorrhage, particularly if prematurity is in combination with antenatal infections or postnatal respiratory disorders. There is, however, still a lot that is not known about platelets in the newborn. Such information is critical to improving the standard of care, intervention, and therapy.

Acknowledgements

This work was supported in part by NIH grant R01 NR011209-08.

Conflict of interest

The authors declare that they have no conflict of interest.

Author details

Ijeoma Esiaba[1,2], Iman Mousselli[3], Giulia M. Faison[4], Danilyn M. Angeles[3] and Danilo S. Boskovic[1,5*]

1 Department of Earth and Biological Sciences, School of Medicine, Loma Linda University, Loma Linda, CA, United States

2 Department of Biochemistry, School of Medicine, Babcock University, Ilishan-Remo, Ogun State, Nigeria

3 Division of Physiology, Department of Basic Sciences, School of Medicine, Loma Linda University, Loma Linda, CA, United States

4 Division of Neonatology, Department of Pediatrics, School of Medicine, Loma Linda University, Loma Linda, CA, United States

5 Division of Biochemistry, Department of Basic Sciences, School of Medicine, Loma Linda University, Loma Linda, CA, United States

*Address all correspondence to: dboskovic@llu.edu

IntechOpen

References

[1] Harrison P. Platelet function analysis. Blood Reviews. 2005;**19**:111-123. DOI: 10.1016/j.blre.2004.05.002

[2] Leslie M. Beyond clotting: The powers of platelets. Science. 2010;**328**(5978):562-564. DOI: 10.1126/science.328.5978.562

[3] Storti F, Kempen THS, Vosse FN. A continuum model for platelet plug formation and growth. International Journal of Numerical Methods in Biomedical Engineering. 2014;**30**(6):634-658. DOI: 10.1002/cnm.2623

[4] Hou Y, Carrim N, Wang Y, Gallant RC, Marshall A, Ni H. Platelets in hemostasis and thrombosis: Novel mechanisms of fibrinogen-independent platelet aggregation and fibronectin-mediated protein wave of hemostasis. Journal of Biomedical Research. 2015;**29**(6): 437-444. DOI: 10.7555/JBR.29.20150121

[5] Muthard RW, Welsh JD, Brass LF, Diamond SL. Fibrin, γ'-fibrinogen, and trans-clot pressure gradient control hemostatic clot growth during human blood flow over a collagen/tissue factor wound. Arteriosclerosis, Thrombosis, and Vascular Biology. 2015;**35**(3):645-654. DOI: 10.1161/ATVBAHA.114.305054

[6] Colace T, Muthard R, Diamond SL. Thrombus growth and embolism on tissue factor-bearing collagen surfaces under flow: Role of thrombin with and without fibrin. Arteriosclerosis, Thrombosis, and Vascular Biology. 2012;**32**(6):1466-1476. DOI: 10.1161/ATVBAHA.112.249789

[7] Manco-Johnson MJ. Development of hemostasis in the fetus and neonate. Thrombosis Research. 2007;**119**:S4-S5. DOI: 10.1016/s0049-3848(07)70004-x

[8] Haley KM, Recht M, McCarty OJT. Neonatal platelets: Mediators of primary hemostasis in the developing hemostatic system. Pediatric Research. 2014;**76**(3):230-237. DOI: 10.1038/pr.2014.87

[9] Boulaftali Y, Hess PR, Getz TM, Cholka A, Stolla M, Mackman N, et al. Platelet ITAM signaling is critical for vascular integrity in inflammation. Journal of Clinical Investigation. 2013;**123**(2):908-916. DOI: 10.1172/jci65154

[10] Kollmann TR, Kampmann B, Mazmanian SK, Marchant A, Levy O. Protecting the newborn and young infant from infectious diseases: Lessons from immune ontogeny. Immunity. 2017;**46**(3):350-363. DOI: 10.1016/j.immuni.2017.03.009

[11] Hallevi H, Walker KC, Kasam M, Bornstein N, Grotta JC, Savitz SI. Inflammatory response to intraventricular hemorrhage: Time course, magnitude and effect of t-PA. Journal of the Neurological Sciences. 2012;**315**(1-2):93-95. DOI: 10.1016/j.jns.2011.11.019

[12] Dani C, Cecchi A, Bertini G. Role of oxidative stress as physiopathologic factor in the preterm infant. Minerva Pediatrica. 2004;**56**(4):381-394

[13] Nurden AT. Platelets, inflammation and tissue regeneration. Thrombosis and Haemostasis. 2011;**105**(99):S13-S33. DOI: 10.1160/THS10-11-0720

[14] Kaushansky K. Historical review: Megakaryopoiesis and thrombopoiesis. Blood. 2008;**111**(3):981-986. DOI: 10.1182/blood-2007-05-088500

[15] Andres O, Schulze H, Speer CP. Platelets in neonates: Central mediators in haemostasis, antimicrobial defence and inflammation. Thrombosis and Haemostasis. 2015;**113**(1):3-12. DOI: 10.1160/TH14-05-0476

[16] Liu Z-J, Hoffmeister KM, Hu Z, Mager DE, Ait-Oudhia S, Debrincat MA, et al. Expansion of the neonatal platelet mass is achieved via an extension of platelet lifespan. Blood. 2014;**123**(22):3381-3389. DOI: 10.1182/blood-2013-06-508200

[17] Watts TL, Murray NA, Roberts IAG. Thrombopoietin has a primary role in the regulation of platelet production in preterm babies. Pediatric Research. 1999;**46**(1):28-32. DOI: 10.1203/00006450-199907000-00005

[18] Murray NA, Watts TL, Roberts IA. Thrombopoietin in the fetus and neonate. Early Human Development. 2000;**59**(1):1-12. DOI: 10.1016/S0378-3782(00)00078-5

[19] Del Vecchio A, Motta M, Romagnoli C. Neonatal platelet function. Clinics in Perinatology. 2015;**42**(3):625-638. DOI: 10.1016/j.clp.2015.04.015

[20] Brass L. Understanding and evaluating platelet function. Hematology. American Society of Hematology. Education Program. 2010;**2010**(1):387-396. DOI: 10.1182/asheducation-2010.1.387

[21] Weyrich AS, Dixon DA, Pabla R, Elstad MR, McIntyre TM, Prescott SM, et al. Signal-dependent translation of a regulatory protein, Bcl-3, in activated human platelets. Proceedings of the National Academy of Sciences of the United States of America. 1998;**95**(10):5556-5561. DOI: 10.1073/pnas.95.10.5556

[22] Golebiewska EM, Poole AW. Platelet secretion: From haemostasis to wound healing and beyond. Blood Reviews. 2015;**29**(3):153-162. DOI: 10.1016/j.blre.2014.10.003

[23] Zarbock A, Polanowska-Grabowska RK, Ley K. Platelet-neutrophil-interactions: Linking hemostasis and inflammation. Blood Reviews. 2007;**21**(2):99-111. DOI: 10.1016/j.blre.2006.06.001

[24] Rondina MT, Weyrich AS, Zimmerman GA. Platelets as cellular effectors of inflammation in vascular diseases. Circulation Research. 2013;**112**(11):1506-1519. DOI: 10.1161/circresaha.113.300512

[25] Ogedegbe HO. An overview of hemostasis. Laboratory Medicine. 2002;**33**(12):948-953. DOI: 10.1092/QWJQLR8ELGL6X32H

[26] Heemskerk JW, Bevers EM, Lindhout T. Platelet activation and blood coagulation. Thrombosis and Haemostasis. 2002;**88**(2):186-193. DOI: 10.1055/s-0037-1613209

[27] Cox D, Kerrigan SW, Watson SP. Platelets and the innate immune system: Mechanisms of bacterial-induced platelet activation. Journal of Thrombosis and Haemostasis. 2011;**9**(6):1097-1107. DOI: 10.1111/j.1538-7836.2011.04264.x

[28] Lentz BR. Exposure of platelet membrane phosphatidylserine regulates blood coagulation. Progress in Lipid Research. 2003;**42**(5):423-438. DOI: 10.1016/S0163-7827(03)00025-0

[29] George JN. Platelets. Lancet. 2000;**355**(9214):1531-1539. DOI: 10.1016/S0140-6736(00)02175-9

[30] Kuhle S, Male C, Mitchell L. Developmental hemostasis: Pro- and anticoagulant systems during childhood. Seminars in Thrombosis and Hemostasis. 2003;**29**(4):329-337. DOI: 10.1055/s-2003-42584

[31] Brass LF. Thrombin and platelet activation. Chest. 2003;**124**(3 Suppl): 18S-25S. DOI: 10.1378/chest.124.3_suppl.18S

[32] Mann K, Brummel-Ziedins K. Normal Coagulation: DTIC Document.2014

[33] Rhee J-S, Black M, Schubert U, Fischer S, Morgenstern E, Hammes H-P, et al. The functional role of blood platelet components in angiogenesis. Thrombosis and Haemostasis. 2004;**92**(2):394-402. DOI: 10.1160/TH03-04-0213

[34] Walsh TG, Metharom P, Berndt MC. The functional role of platelets in the regulation of angiogenesis. Platelets. 2015;**26**(3):199-211. DOI: 10.3109/09537104.2014.909022

[35] Italiano JE, Richardson JL, Patel-Hett S, Battinelli E, Zaslavsky A, Short S, et al. Angiogenesis is regulated by a novel mechanism: Pro- and antiangiogenic proteins are organized into separate platelet α granules and differentially released. Blood. 2008;**111**(3):1227-1233. DOI: 10.1182/blood-2007-09-113837

[36] Bambace NM, Holmes CE. The platelet contribution to cancer progression. Journal of Thrombosis and Haemostasis. 2011;**9**(2):237-249. DOI: 10.1111/j.1538-7836.2010.04131.x

[37] Lacoste B, Gu C. Control of cerebrovascular patterning by neural activity during postnatal development. Mechanisms of Development. 2015;**138**(Pt 1):43-49. DOI: 10.1016/j.mod.2015.06.003

[38] Carr R. Neutrophil production and function in newborn infants. British Journal of Haematology. 2000;**110**(1):18-28. DOI: 10.1046/j.1365-2141.2000.01992.x

[39] Karenberg K, Hudalla H, Frommhold D. Leukocyte recruitment in preterm and term infants. Molecular and Cellular Pediatrics. 2016;**3**(1):35. DOI: 10.1186/s40348-016-0063-5

[40] Kolaczkowska E, Kubes P. Neutrophil recruitment and function in health and inflammation. Nature Reviews Immunology. 2013;**13**(3):159-175. DOI: 10.1038/nri3399

[41] Mauler M, Seyfert J, Haenel D, Seeba H, Guenther J, Stallmann D, et al. Platelet-neutrophil complex formation—A detailed in vitro analysis of murine and human blood samples. Journal of Leukocyte Biology. 2016;**99**(5):781-789. DOI: 10.1189/jlb.3TA0315-082R

[42] Etulain J, Negrotto S, Carestia A, Pozner RG, Romaniuk MA, D'Atri LP, et al. Acidosis downregulates platelet haemostatic functions and promotes neutrophil proinflammatory responses mediated by platelets. Thrombosis and Haemostasis. 2012;**107**(1):99-110. DOI: 10.1160/th11-06-0443

[43] Konstantopoulos K, Neelamegham S, Burns AR, Hentzen E, Kansas GS, Snapp KR. Venous levels of shear support neutrophil-platelet adhesion and neutrophil aggregation in blood via P-selectin and beta2-integrin. Circulation. 1998;**98**(9):873-882. DOI: 10.1161/01.cir.98.9.873

[44] Polanowska-Grabowska R, Wallace K, Field JJ, Chen L, Marshall MA, Figler R, et al. P-selectin–mediated platelet-neutrophil aggregate formation activates neutrophils in mouse and human sickle cell disease. Arteriosclerosis, Thrombosis, and Vascular Biology. 2010;**30**(12):2392-2399. DOI: 10.1161/ATVBAHA.110.211615

[45] Zuchtriegel G, Uhl B, Puhr-Westerheide D, Pörnbacher M, Lauber K, Krombach F, et al. Platelets guide leukocytes to their sites of extravasation. PLoS Biology. 2016;**14**(5):e1002459. DOI: 10.1371/journal.pbio.1002459

[46] Kornerup KN, Salmon GP, Pitchford SC, Liu WL, Page CP. Circulating platelet-neutrophil complexes are important for subsequent neutrophil activation and migration. Journal of Applied Physiology. 2010;**109**(3):758-767. DOI: 10.1152/japplphysiol.01086.2009

[47] Murray NA, Watts TL, Roberts IA. Endogenous thrombopoietin levels and effect of recombinant human thrombopoietin on megakaryocyte precursors in term and preterm babies. Pediatric Research. 1998;**43**(1):148-151. DOI: 10.1203/00006450-199801000-00023

[48] Sola MC, Juul SE, Meng YG, Garg S, Sims P, Calhoun DA, et al. Thrombopoietin (Tpo) in the fetus and neonate. Early Human Development. 1999;**53**(3):239-250. DOI: 10.1016/ S0378-3782(98)00077-2

[49] Ferrer-Marin F, Stanworth S, Josephson C, Sola-Visner M. Distinct differences in platelet production and function between neonates and adults: Implications for platelet transfusion practice. Transfusion. 2013;**53**(11): 2814-2821. DOI: 10.1111/trf.12343

[50] Murray NA, Roberts IA. Circulating megakaryocytes and their progenitors (BFU-MK and CFU-MK) in term and pre-term neonates. British Journal of Haematology. 1995;**89**(1):41-46. DOI: 10.1111/j.1365-2141.1995.tb08913.x

[51] Clapp DW, Baley JE, Gerson SL. Gestational age-dependent changes in circulating hematopoietic stem cells in newborn infants. The Journal of Laboratory and Clinical Medicine. 1989;**113**(4):422-427

[52] Saving K, Aldag J, Jennings D, Caughey B, Regan M, Powers W. Electron-microscopic characterization of neonatal platelet ultrastructure— Effects of sampling techniques. Thrombosis Research. 1991;**61**(1):65-80. DOI: 10.1016/0049-3848(91)90169-w

[53] Saving KL, Jennings DE, Aldag JC, Caughey RC. Platelet ultrastructure of high-risk premature-infants. Thrombosis Research. 1994;**73**(6):371-384. DOI: 10.1016/0049-3848(94)90039-6

[54] Gruel Y, Boizard B, Daffos F, Forestier F, Caen J, Wautier JL. Determination of platelet antigens and glycoproteins in the human fetus. Blood. 1986;**68**(2):488-492

[55] Israels SJ, Odaibo FS, Robertson C, McMillan EM, McNicol A. Deficient thromboxane synthesis and response in platelets from premature infants. Pediatric Research. 1997;**41**(2):218-223. DOI: 10.1203/00006450-199702000-00011

[56] Corby DG, O'Barr TP. Decreased alpha-adrenergic receptors in newborn platelets: Cause of abnormal response to epinephrine. Developmental Pharmacology and Therapeutics. 1981;**2**(4):215-225

[57] Mankin P, Maragos J, Akhand M, Saving KL. Imparied platelet— Dense granule release in neonates. Journal of Pediatric Hematology/ Oncology. 2000;**22**(2):143-147. DOI: 10.1097/00043426-200003000-00012

[58] Wasiluk A, Mantur M, Kemona-Chetnik I, Szczepanski M, Warda J, Bochenko-Luczynska J. Does prematurity affect thrombocytopoiesis? Platelets. 2007;**18**(6):424-427. DOI: 10.1080/09537100701206816

[59] Sola-Visner M. Platelets in the neonatal period: Developmental differences in platelet production, function, and hemostasis and the potential impact of therapies. Hematology. American Society of Hematology. Education Program. 2012;**2012**:506-511. DOI: 10.1182/ asheducation-2012.1.506

[60] Saxonhouse MA, Sola MC, Pastos KM, Ignatz ME, Hutson AD, Christensen RD, et al. Reticulated platelet percentages in term and preterm neonates. Journal of Pediatric Hematology/Oncology. 2004;**26**(12):797-802

[61] Shenkman B, Linder N, Savion N, Tamarin I, Dardik R, Kennet G, et al. Increased neonatal platelet deposition on subendothelium under flow conditions: The role of plasma von Willebrand factor. Pediatric Research. 1999;**45**(2):270-275. DOI: 10.1203/00006450-199902000-00019

[62] Linder N, Shenkman B, Levin E, Sirota L, Vishne T, Tamarin I, et al. Deposition of whole blood platelets on extracellular matrix under flow conditions in preterm infants. Archives of Disease in Childhood. Fetal and Neonatal Edition. 2002;**86**(2):F127-F130. DOI: 10.1136/fn.86.2.F127

[63] Katz JA, Moake JL, McPherson PD, Weinstein MJ, Moise KJ, Carpenter RJ, et al. Relationship between human development and disappearance of unusually large von Willebrand factor multimers from plasma. Blood. 1989;**73**(7):1851-1858

[64] Weinstein MJ, Blanchard R, Moake JL, And EV, Moise K. Fetal and neonatal von Willebrand factor (vWF) is unusually large and similar to the vWF in patients with thrombotic thrombocytopenic purpura. British Journal of Haematology. 1989;**72**(1):68-72. DOI: 10.1111/j.1365-2141.1989.tb07654.x

[65] Bernhard H, Rosenkranz A, Novak M, Leschnik B, Petritsch M, Rehak T, et al. No differences in support of thrombin generation by neonatal or adult platelets. Hämostaseologie. 2009;**29**(Suppl 1):S94-S97

[66] Bernhard H, Rosenkranz A, Petritsch M, Kofeler H, Rehak T, Novak M, et al. Phospholipid content, expression and support of thrombin generation of neonatal platelets. Acta Paediatrica. 2009;**98**(2):251-255. DOI: 10.1111/j.1651-2227.2008.01075.x

[67] Michelson AD, Rajasekhar D, Bednarek FJ, Barnard MR. Platelet and platelet-derived microparticle surface factor V/Va binding in whole blood: Differences between neonates and adults. Thrombosis and Haemostasis. 2000;**84**(4):689-694. DOI: 10.1055/s-0037-1614088

[68] Israels SJ, Daniels M, McMillan EM. Deficient collagen-induced activation in the newborn platelet. Pediatric Research. 1990;**27**(4Pt 1):337-343. DOI: 10.1203/00006450-199004000-00004

[69] Sitaru AG, Holzhauer S, Speer CP, Singer D, Obergfell A, Walter U, et al. Neonatal platelets from cord blood and peripheral blood. Platelets. 2005;**16**(3-4):203-210. DOI: 10.1080/09537100400016862

[70] Rajasekhar D, Barnard MR, Bednarek FJ, Michelson AD. Platelet hyporeactivity in very low birth weight neonates. Thrombosis and Haemostasis. 1997;**77**(5):1002-1007. DOI: 10.1055/s-0038-1656093

[71] Bednarek FJ, Bean S, Barnard MR, Frelinger AL, Michelson AD. The platelet hyporeactivity of extremely low birth weight neonates is age-dependent. Thrombosis Research. 2009;**124**(1):42-45. DOI: 10.1016/j.thromres.2008.10.004

[72] Israels SJ, Rand ML, Michelson AD. Neonatal platelet function. Seminars in Thrombosis and Hemostasis. 2003;**29**(4):363-371. DOI: 10.1055/s-2003-42587

[73] Schlagenhauf A, Schweintzger S, Birner-Gruenberger R, Leschnik B, Muntean W. Newborn platelets: Lower levels of protease-activated receptors cause hypoaggregability to thrombin. Platelets. 2010;**21**(8):641-647. DOI: 10.3109/09537104.2010.504869

[74] Schlagenhauf A, Schweintzger S, Birner-Grünberger R, Leschnik B, Muntean W. Comparative evaluation of PAR1, GPIb-IX-V, and integrin αIIbβ3 levels in cord and adult platelets.

Hämostaseologie. 2010;**30**(4a, Suppl 1): S164-S167

[75] Revel-Vilk S. The conundrum of neonatal coagulopathy. Hematology. American Society of Hematology. Education Program;**2012**:450-454. DOI: 10.1182/asheducation-2012.1.450

[76] Del Vecchio A, Stronati M, Franco C, Christensen RD. Bi-directional activation of inflammation and coagulation in septic neonates. Early Human Development. 2014;**90**:S22-S25. DOI: 10.1016/S0378-3782(14)70008-8

[77] Kalagiri RR, Choudhury S, Carder T, Govande V, Beeram MR, Uddin MN. Neonatal Thrombocytopenia as a consequence of maternal preeclampsia. AJP Reports. 2016;**06**(01):e42-e47. DOI: 10.1055/s-0035-1565923

[78] Burrows RF, Andrew M. Neonatal thrombocytopenia in the hypertensive disorders of pregnancy. Obstetrics and Gynecology. 1990;**76**(2):234-238

[79] Kumar S, Haricharan K. Neonatal thrombocytopenia associated with gestational hypertension, preeclampsia and eclampsia: A case-control study. International Journal of Contemporary Pediatrics. 2016;**3**(1):16-21. DOI: 10.18203/2349-3291.ijcp20151385

[80] Strauss T, Maayan-Metzger A, Simchen MJ, Morag I, Shenkmean B, Kuint J, et al. Impaired platelet function in neonates born to mothers with diabetes or hypertension during pregnancy. Klinische Pädiatrie. 2010;**222**(3):154-157. DOI: 10.1055/s-0030-1249092

[81] Bhat YR, Cherian CS. Neonatal thrombocytopenia associated with maternal pregnancy induced hypertension. Indian Journal of Pediatrics. 2008;**75**(6):571-573. DOI: 10.1007/s12098-008-0110-x

[82] Pritchard JA, Cunningham FG, Pritchard SA, Mason RA. How often does maternal preeclampsia-eclampsia incite thrombocytopenia in the fetus? Obstetrics and Gynecology. 1987;**69** (3Pt 1):292-295

[83] Kuhne T, Ryan G, Blanchette V, Semple JW, Hornstein A, Mody M, et al. Platelet-surface glycoproteins in healthy and preeclamptic mothers and their newborn infants. Pediatric Research. 1996;**40**(6):876-880. DOI: 10.1203/00006450-199612000-00018

[84] Yang J, Zhang H, Niu J, Mu X, Zhang X, Liu Y, et al. Impact of preeclampsia on megakaryocytopoesis and platelet homeostasis of preterm infants. Platelets. 2016;**27**(2):123-127. DOI: 10.3109/09537104.2015.1048213

[85] Roberts I, Murray NA. Neonatal thrombocytopenia: Causes and management. Archives of Disease in Childhood. Fetal and Neonatal Edition. 2003;**88**(5):F359-F364. DOI: 10.1136/fn.88.5.F359

[86] Hutter D, Kingdom J, Jaeggi E. Causes and mechanisms of intrauterine hypoxia and its impact on the fetal cardiovascular system: A review. International Journal of Pediatrics. 2010;**2010**:401323. DOI: 10.1155/2010/401323

[87] Cottrell MB, Jackson CW, McDonald TP. Hypoxia increases erythropoiesis and decreases thrombocytopoiesis in mice: A comparison of two mouse strains. Proceedings of the Society for Experimental Biology and Medicine. 1991;**197**(3):261-267. DOI: 10.3181/00379727-197-43253

[88] Block-Abraham DM, Turan OM, Doyle LE, Kopelman JN, Atlas RO, Jenkins CB, et al. First-trimester risk factors for preeclampsia development in women initiating aspirin by 16 weeks of gestation. Obstetrics and Gynecology. 2014;**123**(3):611-617. DOI: 10.1097/AOG.0000000000000118

[89] Roberge S, Odibo AO, Bujold E. Aspirin for the prevention of preeclampsia and intrauterine growth restriction. Clinics in Laboratory Medicine. 2016;**36**(2):319-329. DOI: 10.1016/j.cll.2016.01.013

[90] Ferreira PMF, Gagliano-Juca T, Zaminelli T, Sampaio MF, Blackler RW, Trevisan MD, et al. Acetylsalicylic acid daily vs acetylsalicylic acid every 3 days in healthy volunteers: Effect on platelet aggregation, gastric mucosa, and prostaglandin E-2 synthesis. Journal of Clinical Pharmacology. 2016;**56**(7): 862-868. DOI: 10.1002/jcph.685

[91] Fitzgerald GA. Mechanisms of platelet activation—Thromboxane-a2 as an amplifying signal for other agonists. The American Journal of Cardiology. 1991;**68**(7):B11-B15. DOI: 10.1016/0002-9149(91)90379-y

[92] Dasari R, Narang A, Vasishta K, Garewal G. Effect of maternal low dose aspirin on neonatal platelet function. Indian Pediatrics. 1998;**35**:507-512

[93] Louden K, Pipkin FB, Heptinstall S, Fox S, Tuohy P, O'Callaghan C, et al. Neonatal platelet reactivity and serum thromboxane B2production in whole blood: The effect of maternal low dose aspirin. British Journal of Obstetrics and Gynaecology. 1994;**101**(3):203-208. DOI: 10.1111/j.1471-0528.1994.tb13110.x

[94] Leonhardt A, Bernert S, Watzer B, Schmitz-Ziegler G, Seyberth HW. Low-dose aspirin in pregnancy: Maternal and neonatal aspirin concentrations and neonatal prostanoid formation. Pediatrics. 2003;**111**(1):e77-e81. DOI: 10.1542/peds.111.1.e77

[95] Bleyer WA, Breckenridge RT. Studies on the detection of adverse drug reactions in the newborn: II. The effects of prenatal aspirin on newborn hemostasis. Journal of the American Medical Association. 1970;**213**(12):2049-2053. DOI: 10.1001/jama.1970.03170380023004

[96] Hammers AL, Sanchez-Ramos L, Kaunitz AM. Antenatal exposure to indomethacin increases the risk of severe intraventricular hemorrhage, necrotizing enterocolitis, and periventricular leukomalacia: A systematic review with metaanalysis. American Journal of Obstetrics and Gynecology. 2015;**212**(4):505.e1. DOI: 10.1016/j.ajog.2014.10.1091

[97] Rhee E, Beiswenger T, Oguejiofor CE, James AH. The effects of magnesium sulfate on maternal and fetal platelet aggregation. The Journal of Maternal-Fetal & Neonatal Medicine. 2012;**25**(5):478-483. DOI: 10.3109/14767058.2011.584087

[98] Brown RE, Rimsza LM, Pastos K, Young L, Saxonhouse MA, Bailey M, et al. Effects of sepsis on neonatal thrombopoiesis. Pediatric Research. 2008;**64**(4):399-404. DOI: 10.1203/PDR.0b013e318181ad49

[99] Finkelstein Y, Shenkman B, Sirota L, Vishne TH, Dardik R, Varon D, et al. Whole blood platelet deposition on extracellular matrix under flow conditions in preterm neonatal sepsis. European Journal of Pediatrics. 2002;**161**(5):270-274. DOI: 10.1007/s00431-002-0938-4

[100] Kara S, Emeksiz Z, Alioğlu B, Dallar Bilge Y. Effects of neonatal sepsis on thrombocyte tests. The Journal of Maternal-Fetal & Neonatal Medicine. 2016;**29**(9):1406-1408. DOI: 10.3109/14767058.2015.1049523

[101] Sitaru AG, Speer CR, Holzhauer S, Obergfell A, Walter U, Grossmann R. Chorioamnionitis is associated with increased CD40L expression on cord blood platelets. Thrombosis and Haemostasis. 2005;**94**(6):1219-1223. DOI: 10.1160/th05-02-0127

[102] Sheffield MJ, Lambert DK, Henry E, Christensen RD. Effect of ampicillin on the bleeding time of neonatal intensive care unit patients. Journal of

Perinatology. 2010;**30**(8):527-530. DOI: 10.1038/jp.2009.192

[103] Sheffield M, Lambert D, Baer V, Henry E, Butler A, Snow G, et al. Effect of ampicillin on bleeding time in very low birth-weight neonates during the first week after birth. Journal of Perinatology. 2011;**31**(7):477-480. DOI: 10.1038/jp.2010.154

[104] Rennie JM, Doyle J, Cooke RW. Early administration of indomethacin to preterm infants. Archives of Disease in Childhood. 1986;**61**(3):233-238. DOI: 10.1136/adc.61.3.233

[105] Corazza MS, Davis RF, Merritt TA, Bejar R, Cvetnic W. Prolonged bleeding time in preterm infants receiving indomethacin for patent ductus arteriosus. The Journal of Pediatrics. 1984;**105**(2):292-296. DOI: 10.1016/S0022-3476(84)80135-3

[106] Friedman Z, Whitman V, Maisels MJ, Berman W Jr, Marks KH, Vesell ES. Indomethacin disposition and indomethacin-induced platelet dysfunction in premature infants. Journal of Clinical Pharmacology. 1978;**18**(5-6):272-279. DOI: 10.1002/j.1552-4604.1978.tb02446.x

[107] Maher P, Lane B, Ballard R, Piecuch R, Clyman RI. Does indomethacin cause extension of intracranial hemorrhages: A preliminary study. Pediatrics. 1985;75(3):497-500

[108] Sheffield MJ, Schmutz N, Lambert DK, Henry E, Christensen RD. Ibuprofen lysine administration to neonates with a patent ductus arteriosus: Effect on platelet plug formation assessed by in vivo and in vitro measurements. Journal of Perinatology. 2009;**29**(1):39-43. DOI: 10.1038/jp.2008.122

[109] Tanriverdi S, Koroglu OA, Uygur O, Balkan C, Yalaz M, Kultursay N. The effect of inhaled nitric oxide therapy on thromboelastogram in newborns with persistent pulmonary hypertension. European Journal of Pediatrics. 2014;**173**(10):1381-1385. DOI: 10.1007/s00431-014-2325-3

[110] Cheung P-Y, Salas E, Schulz R, Radomski MW. Nitric oxide and platelet function: Implications for neonatology. Seminars in Perinatology. 1997;**21**(5):409-417. DOI: 10.1016/S0146-0005(97)80006-7

[111] George TN, Johnson KJ, Bates JN, Segar JL. The effect of inhaled nitric oxide therapy on bleeding time and platelet aggregation in neonates. The Journal of Pediatrics. 1998;**132**(4):731-734. DOI: 10.1016/S0022-3476(98)70370-1

[112] Watala C, Chudzik A, Tchorzewski H, Gwozdzinski K. Impaired action of nitric oxide on blood platelets in premature newborns. Archives of Medical Science. 2008;**4**(3):315-323

[113] Kannar V, Deepthi A, Kumar MLH, Junjegowda K, Mariyappa N. Effect of gestational age, prematurity and birth asphyxia on platelet indices in neonates. Journal of Clinical Neonatology. 2014;**3**(3):144-147. DOI: 10.4103/2249-4847.140399

[114] Wasiluk A, Dabrowska M, Osada J, Jasinska E, Laudanski T, Redzko S. Platelet indices in SGA newborns. Advanced Medical Science. 2011;**56**(2):361-365. DOI: 10.2478/v10039-011-0030-2

[115] Panova-Noeva M, Schulz A, Hermanns MI, Grossmann V, Pefani E, Spronk HMH, et al. Sex-specific differences in genetic and nongenetic determinants of mean platelet volume: Results from the Gutenberg Health Study. Blood. 2016;**127**(2):251-259. DOI: 10.1182/blood-2015-07-660308

[116] Ekin A, Gezer C, Kulhan G, Avci ME, Taner CE. Can platelet count and mean platelet volume during the first

trimester of pregnancy predict preterm premature rupture of membranes? The Journal of Obstetrics and Gynaecology Research. 2015;**41**(1):23-28. DOI: 10.1111/jog.12484

[117] Canpolat FE, Yurdakok M, Armangil D, Yigit S. Mean platelet volume in neonatal respiratory distress syndrome. Pediatrics International. 2009;**51**(2):314-316. DOI: 10.1111/j.1442-200X.2009.02820.x

[118] Aly H, El Beshlawy A, Badrawi N, Mohsen L, Mansour E, Ramy N, et al. Thrombopoietin level is increased in the serum of asphyxiated neonates: A prospective controlled study. Journal of Perinatology. 2005;**25**(5):320-324. DOI: 10.1038/sj.jp.7211287

[119] Christensen RD, Baer VL, Yaish HM. Thrombocytopenia in late preterm and term neonates after perinatal asphyxia. Transfusion. 2015;**55**(1): 187-196. DOI: 10.1111/trf.12777

[120] Brus F, van Oeveren W, Okken A, Oetomo SB. Number and activation of circulating polymorphonuclear leukocytes and platelets are associated with neonatal respiratory distress syndrome severity. Pediatrics. 1997;**99**(5):672-680. DOI: 10.1542/peds.99.5.672

[121] Ballin A, Koren G, Kohelet D, Burger R, Greenwald M, Bryan AC, et al. Reduction of platelet counts induced by mechanical ventilation in newborn infants. The Journal of Pediatrics. 1987;**111**(3):445-449. DOI: 10.1016/S0022-3476(87)80477-8

[122] Postma S, Emara M, Obaid L, Johnson ST, Bigam DL, Cheung PY. Temporal platelet aggregatory function in hypoxic newborn piglets reoxygenated with 18%, 21%, and 100% oxygen. Shock. 2007;**27**(4):448-454. DOI: 10.1097/01.shk.0000245028.47106.92

[123] Boutaybi N, Razenberg F, Smits-Wintjens V, van Zwet EW, Rijken M, Steggerda S, et al. Neonatal thrombocytopenia after perinatal asphyxia treated with hypothermia: A retrospective case control study. International Journal of Pediatrics. 2014;**2014**:760654. DOI: 10.1155/2014/760654

[124] Oncel MY, Erdeve O, Calisici E, Oguz SS, Canpolat FE, Uras N, et al. The effect of whole-body cooling on hematological and coagulation parameters in asphyxic newborns. Pediatric Hematology and Oncology. 2013;**30**(3):246-252. DOI: 10.3109/08880018.2013.771240

[125] Robinson TM, Kickler TS, Walker LK, Ness P, Bell W. Effect of extracorporeal membrane oxygenation on platelets in newborns. Critical Care Medicine. 1993;**21**(7):1029-1034. DOI: 10.1097/00003246-199307000-00018

[126] Cheung PY, Sawicki G, Salas E, Etches PC, Schulz R, Radomski MW. The mechanisms of platelet dysfunction during extracorporeal membrane oxygenation in critically ill neonates. Critical Care Medicine. 2000;**28**(7):2584-2590. DOI: 10.1097/00003246-200007000-00067

[127] Singer M, Deutschman CS, Seymour CW, Shankar-Hari M, Annane D, Bauer M, et al. The third international consensus definitions for sepsis and septic shock (Sepsis-3). Consensus definitions for sepsis and septic shock. Journal of the American Medical Association. 2016;**315**(8): 801-810. DOI: 10.1001/jama.2016.0287

[128] Vieira-de-Abreu A, Campbell RA, Weyrich AS, Zimmerman GA. Platelets: Versatile effector cells in hemostasis, inflammation, and the immune continuum. Seminars in Immunopathology. 2012;**34**(1):5-30. DOI: 10.1007/s00281-011-0286-4

[129] Singer M. The role of mitochondrial dysfunction in sepsis-induced multi-organ failure. Virulence. 2014;**5**(1): 66-72. DOI: 10.4161/viru.26907

[130] Bone RC, Francis PB, Pierce AK. Intravascular coagulation associated with the adult respiratory distress syndrome. The American Journal of Medicine. 1976;**61**(5):585-589. DOI: 10.1016/0002-9343(76)90135-2

[131] Thiery-Antier N, Binquet C, Vinault S, Meziani F, Boisramé-Helms J, Quenot J-P, et al. Is thrombocytopenia an early prognostic marker in septic shock? Critical Care Medicine. 2016;**44**(4):764-772. DOI: 10.1097/ccm.0000000000001520

[132] Claushuis TAM, van Vught LA, Scicluna BP, Wiewel MA, Klein Klouwenberg PMC, Hoogendijk AJ, et al. Thrombocytopenia is associated with a dysregulated host response in critically ill sepsis patients. Blood. 2016;**127**(24):3062-3072. DOI: 10.1182/blood-2015-11-680744

[133] de Stoppelaar SF, van't Veer C, Tvd P. The role of platelets in sepsis. Thrombosis and Haemostasis. 2014;**112**(4):666-677. DOI: 10.1160/TH14-02-0126

[134] Deppermann C, Kubes P. Platelets and infection. Seminars in Immunology. 2016;**28**(6):536-545. DOI: 10.1016/j.smim.2016.10.005

[135] Haines NM, Rycus PT, Zwischenberger JB, Bartlett RH, Ündar A. Extracorporeal life support registry report 2008: Neonatal and pediatric cardiac cases. ASAIO Journal. 2009;**55**(1):111-116. DOI: 10.1097/MAT.0b013e318190b6f7

[136] Groom RC, Froebe S, Martin J, Manfra MJ, Cormack JE, Morse C, et al. Update on pediatric perfusion practice in North America: 2005 survey. The Journal of Extra-Corporeal Technology. 2005;**37**(4):343-350

[137] Thiagarajan RR, Laussen PC, Rycus PT, Bartlett RH, Bratton SL. Extracorporeal membrane oxygenation to aid cardiopulmonary resuscitation in infants and children. Circulation. 2007;**116**(15):1693-1700. DOI: 10.1161/CIRCULATIONAHA.106.680678

[138] Zabrocki LA, Brogan TV, Statler KD, Poss WB, Rollins MD, Bratton SL. Extracorporeal membrane oxygenation for pediatric respiratory failure: Survival and predictors of mortality. Critical Care Medicine. 2011;**39**(2):364-370. DOI: 10.1097/CCM.0b013e3181fb7b35

[139] Reed RC, Rutledge JC. Laboratory and clinical predictors of thrombosis and hemorrhage in 29 pediatric extracorporeal membrane oxygenation nonsurvivors. Pediatric and Developmental Pathology. 2010;**13**(5):385-392. DOI: 10.2350/09-09-0704-OA.1

[140] Zwischenberger JB, Nguyen TT, Upp JR Jr, Bush PE, Cox CS Jr, Delosh T, et al. Complications of neonatal extracorporeal membrane oxygenation: Collective experience from the extracorporeal life support organization. The Journal of Thoracic and Cardiovascular Surgery. 1994;**107**(3):838-849

[141] Kim HS, Cheon DY, Ha SO, Han SJ, Kim H-S, Lee SH, et al. Early changes in coagulation profiles and lactate levels in patients with septic shock undergoing extracorporeal membrane oxygenation. Journal of Thoracic Disease. 2018;**10**(3):1418-1430. DOI: 10.21037/jtd.2018.02.28

[142] Fletcher Sandersjöö A, Bartek J, Thelin EP, Eriksson A, Elmi-Terander A, Broman M, et al. Predictors of intracranial hemorrhage in adult patients on extracorporeal membrane oxygenation: An observational cohort study. Journal of Intensive Care.

2017;**5**(1). DOI: 27. DOI: 10.1186/
s40560-017-0223-2

[143] Kreyer S, Muders T, Theuerkauf N,
Spitzhüttl J, Schellhaas T, Schewe J-C,
et al. Hemorrhage under veno-venous
extracorporeal membrane oxygenation
in acute respiratory distress syndrome
patients: A retrospective data
analysis. Journal of Thoracic Disease.
2017;**9**(12):5017-5029. DOI: 10.21037/
jtd.2017.11.05

[144] Lockie CJA, Gillon SA, Barrett NA,
Taylor D, Mazumder A, Paramesh K,
et al. Severe respiratory failure,
extracorporeal membrane oxygenation,
and intracranial hemorrhage. Critical
Care Medicine. 2017;**45**(10):1642-1649.
DOI: 10.1097/CCM.0000000000002579

[145] Oliver WC. Anticoagulation and
coagulation management for ECMO.
Seminars in Cardiothoracic and Vascular
Anesthesia. 2009;**13**(3):154-175. DOI:
10.1177/1089253209347384

[146] Passmore MR, Fung YL, Simonova
G, Foley SR, Diab SD, Dunster KR,
et al. Evidence of altered haemostasis
in an ovine model of venovenous
extracorporeal membrane oxygenation
support. Critical Care. 2017;**21**(1):191.
DOI: 10.1186/s13054-017-1788-9

[147] Lukito P, Wong A, Jing J, Arthur JF,
Marasco SF, Murphy DA, et al.
Mechanical circulatory support is
associated with loss of platelet receptors
glycoprotein Ibα and glycoprotein
VI. Journal of Thrombosis and
Haemostasis. 2016;**14**(11):2253-2260.
DOI: 10.1111/jth.13497

[148] Hawiger J. Formation and
regulation of platelet and fibrin
hemostatic plug. Human Pathology.
1987;**18**(2):111-122. DOI: 10.1016/
S0046-8177(87)80330-1

[149] Ivanciu L, Krishnaswamy S,
Camire RM. Imaging coagulation
reactions in vivo. Thrombosis Research.

2012;**129**(Suppl 2):S54-S56. DOI:
10.1016/j.thromres.2012.02.034

[150] Hase T, Sirajuddin S, Maluso P,
Bangalore R, DePalma L, Sarani B.
Platelet dysfunction in critically ill
patients. Blood Coagulation and
Fibrinolysis. 2017;**28**(6):475-478. DOI:
10.1097/mbc.0000000000000625

[151] Kalbhenn J, Schmidt R, Nakamura
L, Schelling J, Rosenfelder S, Zieger B.
Early diagnosis of acquired von
Willebrand Syndrome (AVWS) is
elementary for clinical practice in
patients treated with ECMO therapy.
Journal of Atherosclerosis and
Thrombosis. 2015;**22**(3):265-271. DOI:
10.5551/jat.27268

[152] Dewanjee MK, Wu SM,
Kapadvanjwala M, De D, Dewanjee S,
Gonzalez L, et al. Emboli from an
extraluminal blood flow hollow fiber
oxygenator with and without an
arterial filter during cardiopulmonary
bypass in a pig model. ASAIO
Journal. 1996;**42**(6):1010-1018. DOI:
10.1097/00002480-199642060-00015

[153] Meyer AD, Gelfond JA, Wiles AA,
Freishtat RJ, Rais-Bahrami K. Platelet-
derived microparticles generated by
neonatal extracorporeal membrane
oxygenation systems. ASAIO Journal.
2015;**61**(1):37-42. DOI: 10.1097/
MAT.0000000000000164

[154] Miyazaki Y, Nomura S, Miyake T,
Kagawa H, Kitada C, Taniguchi H,
et al. High shear stress can initiate both
platelet aggregation and shedding of
procoagulant containing microparticles.
Blood. 1996;**88**(9):3456-3464

[155] Crowther MA, Cook DJ, Meade
MO, Griffith LE, Guyatt GH, Arnold
DM, et al. Thrombocytopenia in
medical-surgical critically ill patients:
Prevalence, incidence, and risk
factors. Journal of Critical Care.
2005;**20**(4):348-353. DOI: 10.1016/j.
jcrc.2005.09.008

[156] Williamson DR, Albert M, Heels-Ansdell D, Arnold DM, Lauzier F, Zarychanski R, et al. Thrombocytopenia in critically ill patients receiving thromboprophylaxis: Frequency, risk factors, and outcomes. Chest. 2013;**144**(4):1207-1215. DOI: 10.1378/chest.13-0121

[157] Abrams D, Baldwin MR, Champion M, Agerstrand C, Eisenberger A, Bacchetta M, et al. Thrombocytopenia and extracorporeal membrane oxygenation in adults with acute respiratory failure: A cohort study. Intensive Care Medicine. 2016;**42**(5):844-852. DOI: 10.1007/s00134-016-4312-9

[158] Lieberman L, Bercovitz RS, Sholapur NS, Heddle NM, Stanworth SJ, Arnold DM. Platelet transfusions for critically ill patients with thrombocytopenia. Blood. 2014;**123**(8):1146-1151. DOI: 10.1182/blood-2013-02-435693

[159] Bembea MM, Annich G, Rycus P, Oldenburg G, Berkowitz I, Pronovost P. Variability in anticoagulation management of patients on extracorporeal membrane oxygenation: An international survey. Pediatric Critical Care Medicine. 2013;**14**(2):E77-E84. DOI: 10.1097/PCC.0b013e31827127e4

[160] Faraoni D, Levy JH. Algorithm-based management of bleeding in patients with extracorporeal membrane oxygenation. Critical Care. 2013;**17**(3):432. DOI: 10.1186/cc12682

[161] Nair P, Hoechter DJ, Buscher H, Venkatesh K, Whittam S, Joseph J, et al. Prospective observational study of hemostatic alterations during adult extracorporeal membrane oxygenation (ECMO) using point-of-care thromboelastometry and platelet aggregometry. Journal of Cardiothoracic and Vascular Anesthesia. 2015;**29**(2):288-296. DOI: 10.1053/j.jvca.2014.06.006

[162] Young G, Yonekawa KE, Nakagawa P, Nugent DJ. Argatroban as an alternative to heparin in extracorporeal membrane oxygenation circuits. Perfusion. 2004;**19**(5):283-288. DOI: 10.1191/0267659104pf759oa

[163] Jyoti A, Maheshwari A, Daniel E, Motihar A, Bhathiwal RS, Sharma D. Bivalirudin in venovenous extracorporeal membrane oxygenation. The Journal of Extra-Corporeal Technology. 2014;**46**(1):94-97

[164] Gray B, Rintoul N. ELSO Guidelines for Cardiopulmonary Extracorporeal Life Support. Version 1.4. Extracorporeal Life Support Organization: Ann Arbor, MI, USA; 2017

[165] Cuker A. Clinical and laboratory diagnosis of heparin-induced thrombocytopenia: An integrated approach. Seminars in Thrombosis and Hemostasis. 2014;**40**(1):106-114. DOI: 10.1055/s-0033-1363461

[166] Schmugge M, Risch L, Huber AR, Benn A, Fischer JE. Heparin-induced thrombocytopenia-associated thrombosis in pediatric intensive care patients. Pediatrics. 2002;**109**(1):E10. DOI: 10.1542/peds.109.1.e10

[167] Klenner AF, Lubenow N, Raschke R, Greinacher A. Heparin-induced thrombocytopenia in children: 12 new cases and review of the literature. Thrombosis and Haemostasis. 2004;**91**(4):719-724. DOI: 10.1160/TH03-09-0571

[168] Risch L, Fischer JE, Herklotz R, Huber AR. Heparin-induced thrombocytopenia in paediatrics: Clinical characteristics, therapy and outcomes. Intensive Care Medicine. 2004;**30**(8):1615-1624. DOI: 10.1007/s00134-004-2315-4

[169] Severin T, Sutor AH. Heparin-induced thrombocytopenia in pediatrics. Seminars in Thrombosis and

Hemostasis. 2001;**27**(3):293-299. DOI: 10.1055/s-2001-15259

[170] Pollak U, Yacobobich J, Tamary H, Dagan O, Manor-Shulman O. Heparin-induced thrombocytopenia and extracorporeal membrane oxygenation: A case report and review of the literature. The Journal of Extra-Corporeal Technology. 2011;**43**(1):5-12

[171] Lee GM, Arepally GM. Heparin-induced thrombocytopenia. Hematology. American Society of Hematology. Education Program. 2013;**2013**(1):668-674. DOI: 10.1182/asheducation-2013.1.668

[172] Warkentin TE. HIT paradigms and paradoxes. Journal of Thrombosis and Haemostasis. 2011;**9**(Suppl 1):105-117. DOI: 10.1111/j.1538-7836.2011.04322.x

[173] Crowther M, Cook D, Guyatt G, Zytaruk N, McDonald E, Williamson D, et al. Heparin-induced thrombocytopenia in the critically ill: Interpreting the 4Ts test in a randomized trial. Journal of Critical Care. 2014;**29**(3):470.e7. DOI: 10.1016/j.jcrc.2014.02.004

[174] Beiderlinden M, Treschan T, Görlinger K, Peters J. Argatroban in extracorporeal membrane oxygenation. Artificial Organs. 2007;**31**(6):461-465. DOI: 10.1111/j.1525-1594.2007.00388.x

[175] Lequier L, Annich G, Al-Ibrahim O, Bembea M, Brodie D, Brogan T. ELSO Anticoagulation Guidelines. Ann Arbor, MI: Extracorporeal Life Support Organization; 2014

[176] Ramasethu J, Luban N. Red blood cell transfusions in the newborn. Seminars in Neonatology. 1999;**4**(1):5-16

[177] Del Vecchio A, Franco C, Petrillo F, D'Amato G. Neonatal transfusion practice: When do neonates need red blood cells or platelets?

American Journal of Perinatology. 2016;**33**(11):1079-1084. DOI: 10.1055/s-0036-1586106

[178] Sola-Visner M, Bercovitz RS. Neonatal platelet transfusions and future areas of research. Transfusion Medicine Reviews. 2016;**304** SI:183-188. DOI: 10.1016/j.tmrv.2016.05.009

[179] Cremer M, Sallmon H, Kling PJ, Buhrer C, Dame C. Thrombocytopenia and platelet transfusion in the neonate. Seminars in Fetal and Neonatal Medicine. 2016;**21**(1):10-18. DOI: 10.1016/j.siny.2015.11.001

[180] Castle V, Andrew M, Kelton J, Giron D, Johnston M, Carter C. Frequency and mechanism of neonatal thrombocytopenia. The Journal of Pediatrics. 1986;**108**(5):749-755. DOI: 10.1016/S0022-3476(86)81059-9

[181] Mehta P, Vasa R, Neumann L, Karpatkin M. Thrombocytopenia in the high-risk infant. The Journal of Pediatrics. 1980;**97**(5):791-794. DOI: 10.1016/S0022-3476(80)80272-1

[182] Christensen RD, Henry E, Wiedmeier SE, Stoddard RA, Sola-Visner MC, Lambert DK, et al. Thrombocytopenia among extremely low birth weight neonates: Data from a multihospital healthcare system. Journal of Perinatology. 2006;**26**(6):348-353. DOI: 10.1038/sj.jp.7211509

[183] Andrew M, Vegh P, Caco C, Kirpalani H, Jefferies A, Ohlsson A, et al. A randomized, controlled trial of platelet transfusions in thrombocytopenic premautre infants. The Journal of Pediatrics. 1993;**123**(2):285-291. DOI: 10.1016/S0022-3476(05)81705-6

[184] Gunnink SF, Vlug R, Fijnvandraat K, van der Bom JG, Stanworth SJ, Lopriore E. Neonatal thrombocytopenia: Etiology, management and outcome. Expert Review of Hematology.

2014;7(3):387-395. DOI: 10.1586/17474086.2014.902301

[185] Resch E, Hinkas O, Urlesberger B, Resch B. Neonatal thrombocytopenia-causes and outcomes following platelet transfusions. European Journal of Pediatrics. 2018;**177**(7):1045-1052. DOI: 10.1007/s00431-018-3153-7

[186] Venkatesh V, Khan R, Curley A, New H, Stanworth S. How we decide when a neonate needs a transfusion. British Journal of Haematology. 2013;**160**(4): 421-433. DOI: 10.1111/bjh.12095

[187] Sparger KA, Assmann SF, Granger S, Winston A, Christensen RD, Widness JA, et al. Platelet transfusion practices among very-low-birth-weight infants. JAMA Pediatrics. 2016;**170**(7):687-694. DOI: 10.1001/jamapediatrics.2016.0507

[188] Cremer M, Weimann A, Schmalisch G, Hammer H, Buhrer C, Dame C. Immature platelet values indicate impaired megakaryopoietic activity in neonatal early-onset thrombocytopenia. Thrombosis and Haemostasis. 2010;**103**(5 SI):1016-1021. DOI: 10.1160/TH09-03-0148

[189] MacQueen BC, Christensen RD, Henry E, Romrell AM, Pysher TJ, Bennett ST, et al. The immature platelet fraction: Creating neonatal reference intervals and using these to categorize neonatal thrombocytopenias. Journal of Perinatology. 2017;**37**(7):834-838. DOI: 10.1038/jp.2017.48

[190] Sparger K, Deschmann E, Sola-Visner M. Platelet transfusions in the neonatal intensive care unit. Clinics in Perinatology. 2015;**42**(3):613-623. DOI: 10.1016/j.clp.2015.04.009

[191] Wiedmeier SE, Henry E, Sola-Visner MC, Christensen RD. Platelet reference ranges for neonates, defined using data from over 47,000 patients in a multihospital healthcare system. Journal of Perinatology. 2009;**29**(2):130-136. DOI: 10.1038/jp.2008.141

[192] Poryo M, Boeckh JC, Gortner L, Zemlin M, Duppre P, Ebrahimi-Fakhari D, et al. Ante-, peri- and postnatal factors associated with intraventricular hemorrhage in very premature infants. Early Human Development. 2018;**116**:1-8. DOI: 10.1016/j.earlhumdev.2017.08.010

[193] Curley A, Stanworth SJ, Willoughby K, Fustolo-Gunnink SF, Venkatesh V, Hudson C, et al. Randomized trial of platelet-transfusion thresholds in neonates. The New England Journal of Medicine. 2019;**380**(3):242-251. DOI: 10.1056/NEJMoa1807320

[194] New HV, Berryman J, Bolton-Maggs PH, Cantwell C, Chalmers EA, Davies T, et al. Guidelines on transfusion for fetuses, neonates and older children. British Journal of Haematology. 2016;**175**(5):784-828. DOI: 10.1111/bjh.14233

[195] Liumbruno G, Bennardello F, Lattanzio A, Piccoli P, Rossetti G, et al. Recommendations for the transfusion of plasma and platelets. Blood Transfusion. 2009;7(2):132-150. DOI: 10.2450/2009.0005-09

[196] Cremer M, Sola-Visner M, Roll S, J osephson CD, Yilmaz Z, Buhrer C, et al. Platelet transfusions in neonates: Practices in the United States vary significantly from those in Austria, Germany, and Switzerland. Transfusion. 2011;**51**(12):2634-2641. DOI: 10.1111/j.1537-2995.2011.03208.x

[197] Josephson CD, Su LL, Christensen RD, Hillyer CD, Castillejo MI, Emory MR, et al. Platelet transfusion practices among neonatologists in the United States and Canada: Results of a survey. Pediatrics. 2009;**123**(1):278-285. DOI: 10.1542/peds.2007-2850

[198] Baer VL, Lambert DK, Henry E, Snow GL, Sola-Visner MC, Christensen RD. Do platelet transfusions in the NICU adversely affect survival? Analysis of 1600 thrombocytopenic

neonates in a multihospital healthcare system. Journal of Perinatology. 2007;**27**(12):790-796. DOI: 10.1038/ sj.jp.7211833

[199] Forman KR, Wong E, Gallagher M, McCarter R, Luban NLC, Massaro AN. Effect of temperature on thromboelastography and implications for clinical use in newborns undergoing therapeutic hypothermia. Pediatric Research. 2014;**75**(5):663-669. DOI: 10.1038/pr.2014.19

[200] Chakkarapani E, Davis J, Thoresen M. Therapeutic hypothermia delays the C-reactive protein response and suppresses white blood cell and platelet count in infants with neonatal encephalopathy. Archives of Disease in Childhood. Fetal and Neonatal Edition. 2014;**99**(6):F485-F463. DOI: 10.1136/ archdischild-2013-305763

[201] Christensen RD, Sheffield MJ, Lambert DK, Baer VL. Effect of therapeutic hypothermia in neonates with hypoxic-ischemic encephalopathy on platelet function. Neonatology. 2012;**101**(2):91-94. DOI: 10.1159/000329818

Chapter 5

Therapeutic Options in Retinopathy of Prematurity

Simona Delia Nicoară

Abstract

Preterm babies may develop retinopathy of prematurity (ROP) in various stages. Most of them regress spontaneously without treatment, and a small proportion develops severe ROP that can lead to visual loss if not treated promptly. Less than 10% of the ROP cases require treatment worldwide. Before 1980, the only treatment for ROP was vitreoretinal surgery for retinal detachment in advanced stages of the disease. Around this time, cryotherapy started to be used in order to ablate the peripheral retina and interrupt the pathogenic chain in ROP, but there were no indications correlated with the severity of the disease. Few years later, cryotherapy was replaced by indirect laser photocoagulation of the nonvascular retina that became the golden standard of treatment for ROP. During the last years, efforts have been made in order to find therapeutic methods to induce the regression of new vessels with minimal side effects. Among these, intravitreal injections of anti-vascular endothelial growth factor (VEGF) became increasingly popular in the treatment of ROP worldwide. Personal experience in treating aggressive posterior ROP (APROP) with laser versus intravitreal anti-VEGF is presented. Intravitreal anti-VEGF proved its superiority in treating APROP as compared to laser, with no systemic and/or local side effects in our series.

Keywords: retinopathy of prematurity, laser, bevacizumab, cryotherapy, blindness

1. Introduction

All high-risk pregnancies are on the rise, and most of them result in a premature birth which is induced either due to maternal factors or fetal factors. Moreover, theoretically there could be more instances where retinopathy of prematurity (ROP) can develop because there has been a lot of development as well as success in management of preterm babies. Progress in neonatal care was associated with higher survival rates of low birth weight and low gestational age newborns.

Retinopathy of prematurity (ROP) is an important threat for the vision of the premature infants, especially for those born at low postconceptional ages (PCAs) and with low birth weights (BWs) [1, 2].

Following progress in neonatal care, the prevalence of ROP is increasing in the developing world, justifying the identification of ROP as a leading cause of visual impairment in children in the developing world, by the World Health Organization (WHO) [1].

In the developed countries, ROP accounts for 4% of childhood blindness, whereas in the developing ones, ROP generates 40% of it [1].

Many preterm babies will develop ROP in various stages. Most of them regress spontaneously without treatment, and a small proportion develops severe ROP that can lead to visual loss if not treated promptly [3]. ROP is one of the few largely preventable causes of visual impairment in children [3–5].

Fortunately, a treatment is available that can significantly reduce the rate of unfavorable outcomes [1]. The early detection of ROP and the prompt treatment are crucial for the prevention of blindness. Currently, there are two therapeutic methods to treat ROP: intravitreal injections with anti-vascular endothelial growth factor (VEGF) agents and indirect laser photocoagulation of the nonvascularized retina [2].

2. Pathophysiology of ROP

During the first 4 months of gestation, the retina has no blood vessels, and it is nourished by the hyaloid vasculature [6].

At 16 weeks, the angioblasts near the hyaloid artery invade the nerve fiber layer, and the first retinal vessels appear at the level of the optic nerve head. They grow progressively toward the periphery, reaching the ora serrata at 36 weeks in the nasal sector and at 40 weeks in the temporal one [6].

The development of the superficial and deep layers of the retinal vasculature depends on the delicate balance between the growth factors which are secreted by the astrocytes and the microglia: vascular endothelial growth factor (VEGF) and insulin growth factor-1 (IGF-1) [6].

During the second half of pregnancy, there is relative intrauterine hypoxia. When premature birth occurs, retinal vessels are not completely developed. Altered oxygen condition is a risk factor for the development of ROP which is a biphasic disease.

The first phase (from the moment of birth to 31- to 32-week postconceptional age) is characterized by relative environmental hyperoxia which leads to the arrest of the normal retinal development [6].

During the second phase (from 32- to 36-week postconceptional age), the retina matures, and its metabolic needs increase. By consequence, it is characterized by relative hypoxia and overexpression of VEGF, IGF-1, and oxidative damage with subsequent new vessel growth and retinal detachment [6].

The association between ROP and the administration of high doses of oxygen was demonstrated for the first time by Patz et al. in 1953 [6].

3. ROP classification

ROP was classified for the first time in 1984 by an international group of experts and updated in 2005. In classifying ROP, three criteria are used: zone, stage, and presence/absence of "plus" disease [7].

Topographically, the retina is divided into three zones. Zone 1 corresponds to a circle centered on the optic disc and with the radius equal to the double distance between the optic disc and the fovea. Zone 2 corresponds to a circle centered on the optic disc with the radius equal to the distance between the optic disc and ora serrata nasally. Zone 3 corresponds to the remaining crescent of the temporal retina up to ora serrata [7].

The stage describes the retinal changes at the limit between the vascular and nonvascular retina. Stage 1 is defined by a demarcation line, stage 2 by a nonvascular (white) ridge, and stage 3 by a vascular (red) ridge. Stage 4a corresponds to peripheral retinal detachment, stage 4b involves also the detachment of the fovea, and stage 5 represents total retinal detachment in an open or closed funnel. "Plus" disease refers to the dilation and irregularity of retinal arteries and veins in the posterior pole, as compared to a standard photograph [7].

Aggressive posterior ROP (APROP) is a subtype of ROP with a very unpredictable and aggressive behavior. It is always located posterior (zone 1 and posterior zone 2), with very severe "plus" disease and with flat neovascularization that progresses rapidly, without getting through the stages described above [7].

The Early Treatment for ROP (ETROP) study reclassified ROP according to the required attitude: type 1, ROP requiring treatment and type 2, ROP requiring closely monitoring.

4. Diagnosis and screening for ROP

Fortunately, it is estimated that less than 10% of the ROP cases require treatment worldwide. More than 90% regress spontaneously [1].

Various screening criteria apply in different countries/regions. For instance, in the USA, the screening criteria updated in 2013 include all infants with BW of 1500 g or less or GA 30 weeks or less.

Heavier and more mature babies are included in the screening at the discretion of the neonatologist, especially if other complications are present: necrotizing enterocolitis, intraventricular hemorrhage, sepsis, and bronchopulmonary dysplasia. According to our national guidelines, all premature newborns with GA of 34 weeks or less or with BW 2000 grams or less are included in the ROP screening.

The first screening should be performed at 4–6 weeks after birth or at PCA 31 weeks whichever is later. When examining a premature infant, one of three situations can be identified: mature retina, immature retinal vascularization, or ROP. ROP screening can be discontinued if retinal vascularization is present in zone 3, without previous zone 1 or zone 2 disease; there is no evidence of prethreshold disease or worse ROP by 50 weeks PCA; there is regressing ROP in zone 3 without abnormal vascular tissue that can reactivate in zone 2 or 3.

ROP screening is made by trained ophthalmologists, using indirect ophthalmoscopy and scleral indentation in order to have access to the retinal periphery. Pupils must be dilated with a mixture of tropicamide 0.5% and phenylephrine 2.5%, and the lids are maintained open with a lid speculum throughout the examination.

5. Prevention and risk factors

The most important factor to prevent ROP is preventing premature birth [6].

The STOP-ROP multicenter study evaluated the risk for prethreshold ROP development in correlation with the oxygen saturation, and it showed no difference between maintaining an oxygen saturation level of 96–99% versus 89–94% [6].

BOOST II study showed a higher survival rate in infants younger than 28 weeks GA with 91–95% oxygen saturation levels but with an increased risk of ROP at this oxygen rate in other studies [6].

6. Treatment of ROP

Before 1980 the only treatment for ROP was vitreoretinal surgery for retinal detachment in advanced stages of the disease. Around this time cryotherapy started to be used in order to ablate the peripheral retina and thus interrupt the pathogenic chain in ROP, but there were no guided indications in correlation with the severity of the disease [6].

CRYO-ROP elaborated a classification of ROP and defined "threshold" disease in which therapy was indicated: 5 contiguous hours or 8 non-contiguous hours of stage 3 ROP with plus disease in zone 1 or 2 [8].

A subsequent study, ETROP investigated whether treatment performed earlier than in threshold disease would further reduce the rate of anatomic unfavorable outcomes. Prethreshold disease was defined as type 1 and type 2 ROP. Clinically, type 1 ROP includes the following categories: zone 1 ROP of any stage with plus, zone 1 stage 3 ROP without plus, and zone 2 stage 2 or 3 disease with plus. In type 2 ROP, the following situations are included: zone 1 stage 1 or 2 without plus or zone 2 stage 3 without plus. ETROP recommends treatment in type 1 ROP and monitoring in type 2 ROP. At 6-year follow-up, the study proved 9% unfavorable structural outcomes in the early treated eyes, as compared to 15% unfavorable structural outcomes in the conventional treatment group. ETROP recommends peripheral laser ablation in type 1 ROP and frequent observation in type 2 ROP.

At this point, ablation of the peripheral retina was made by indirect laser photocoagulation that had replaced cryotherapy [9].

There are several advantages of laser over cryotherapy: laser requires less general anesthesia, it treats easier the posterior ROP, and it is associated with less systemic side effects: apnea, bradycardia, and cardiopulmonary arrest requiring resuscitation. However, ocular complications were reported after extensive indirect diode laser photocoagulation: vitreous hemorrhage, cataract, intraocular inflammation, choroidal effusion, and elevated intraocular pressure [9]. Theoretically, the risk of cataract is very low, given the fact that the infrared radiation that we use is absorbed deep into the choroid and not in the crystalline lens. Vitreous hemorrhage is rather a sign of ROP progression than a complication related to the laser itself.

Parvaresh et al. published the results of transscleral diode laser photocoagulation instead of transpupillary approach and concluded that it is technically easier, especially for retinal periphery and with fewer complications at the level of the anterior segment such as cataract formation [10].

During the last years, efforts have been made in order to find therapeutic methods to induce the regression of new vessels with minimal side effects [10].

Given the role of VEGF in angiogenesis, anti-VEGF administered intravitreally emerged as a promising tool for the treatment of ROP, alongside its use in ischemic retinopathies. Research conducted over the latest two decades proved that VEGF is one of the major factors involved in ROP pathogenesis [10].

VEGF inhibition with subsequent suppression of neovascular disease was proved by several experimental and clinical studies [10].

Clinical studies showed significantly higher levels of VEGF in the vitreous of patients with vasoproliferative ROP [11–13]. Sato et al. analyzed 27 cytokines in the vitreous of ROP eyes and found that VEGF was the most strongly correlated with vascularly active ROP [11]. This study also identified other factors elevated in ROP: fibroblast growth factor (FGF), granulocyte-colony stimulating factor (G-CSF), and granulocyte macrophage-colony stimulating factor (GM-CSF). This observation sustains the participation of an inflammatory response in the complex process of ROP development in addition to known vascular growth factors such as VEGF.

Animal ROP models showed the suppression of the vascular disease following intravitreal anti-VEGF injection [14, 15].

Nonobe et al. injected bevacizumab in the vitreous of five premature infants and showed the marked decrease of aqueous humor concentration of VEGF in four of them. Law et al. injected bevacizumab in 13 eyes of seven premature infants prior to laser or vitrectomy, and they noticed the improvement of the visualization of the retina with no systemic side effects, suggesting the role of anti-VEGF therapy prior these procedures [10].

A retrospective study carried by Lee et al. on 15 premature infants with stage 3 ROP showed the rapid regression of plus disease with more rapid development of normal vessels toward the retinal periphery, with no significant increase in systemic or ocular complications, compared with patients treated with laser photocoagulation [10].

Considerably concerns remain regarding the safety of anti-VEGF treatment in ROP, especially considering the correct dosage, timing of injection, and potential local complications such as infection, lens damage, and effect on the development of the neurosensory retina. Systemic side effects were not reported yet, but concern persists especially regarding the development of the central nervous system.

The Bevacizumab Eliminates the Angiogenic Threat of Retinopathy of Prematurity (BEATROP) study concluded that one doze of bevacizumab 0.625 mg in 0.025 ml had significantly better results in reducing the recurrence rate in zone 1 stage 3 ROP as compared to laser: 6 versus 42%, respectively. However, in posterior zone 2 ROP, the results were similar with intravitreal bevacizumab and laser. An interesting observation was that in some cases treated with intravitreal bevacizumab, late recurrence was noted: 16 ± 4.6 weeks with bevacizumab, as compared to 6.2 ± 5.7 weeks with laser. Therefore, follow-up in anti-VEGF-treated eyes should be performed for longer periods [10].

Erythropoietin (Epo) is another growth factor that was proved to promote angiogenesis in vitro and in animal models. Recombinant Epo (rhEpo) is used to treat anemia in premature infants, as it promotes red blood cell formation. Sato et al. showed significantly elevated levels of Epo in 40 eyes from 27 premature infants with stage 4 ROP [13]. Suk et al. carried out a retrospective study in which he investigated the rhEpo treatment and ROP in 265 patients. The study concluded that high dose and later starting age for rhEpo treatment are risk factors for ROP (the phase of the disease was not taken into account). However, Shah et al. in a retrospective study on 85 patients found no correlation between the rhEpo treatment and the incidence and severity of ROP [16].

Research in the field of angiogenesis led to a number of new ways to prevent ROP progression: targeting the insulin growth factor (IGF-1) pathway and dietary supplementation with omega-3 polyunsaturated fatty acids (PUFAs) [10].

Following preterm birth, serum IGF-1 is substantially reduced due to the interruption of fetal-maternal interaction. Animal models of ROP proved that IGF-1 is essential for vascular growth through interaction with VEGF signaling. Therefore, theoretically, supplementation of IGF-1 during phase 1 ROP would normalize vascular growth and subsequently prevent abnormal vascular proliferation in phase 2 ROP [10].

Omega-3 PUFAs protect against pathologic neovascularization in ROP. They lack from the diet of premature infants because there is no transfer from the mother during the last trimester. Therefore, studies are planned to investigate the potential benefit of supplementing omega-3 PUFA intake in premature infants [10].

Currently, laser photocoagulation of the nonvascular retina remains the only well-established, gold standard therapy to prevent ROP progression toward blindness. There is clinical and experimental research going on in order to add therapeutic strategies meant to improve the prognosis of this potentially blinding disease.

Despite timely treatment, it is estimated that approximately 16% of patients with type 1 ROP develop retinal detachment. The results reported by a large series of cases showed that the reattachment rate following pars plana vitrectomy is correlated with the stage of ROP: 82% for stage 4A, 70% for stage 4B, and 43% for stage

5 ROP. Scleral buckles can also be used for stage 4A ROP. A small case series showed that the association of a scleral buckle to pars plana vitrectomy did not improve the reattachment rate as compared cu PPV alone [10].

Because the therapeutic results in stage 5 ROP are extremely poor, the goal is to screen and treat type 1 ROP before the occurrence of retinal detachment.

In some circumstances, exudative retinal detachment is present, as a result of leakage from the vascular structures. This type of detachment is usually located posterior to the ridge, and it is convex in shape. Favorable results were reported in some of these cases after intravitreal administration of bevacizumab [10].

7. Personal experience in the treatment of aggressive posterior ROP (APROP)

7.1 Background

APROP is a particularly severe form of ROP defined by the following characteristics: posterior location (zone I or posterior zone II), very dilated and tortuous vessels, and development of arteriovenous shunts [17]. The evolution of APROP toward retinal detachment is very rapid, without the stages described in the "classic" form of ROP.

Laser treatment of ROP became available in the Ophthalmology Department ("Iuliu Hatieganu" University of Medicine and Pharmacy from Cluj-Napoca, Romania) in 2006, whereas intravitreal bevacizumab injections started to be used in 2009 (Avastin; Genentech Inc., San Francisco, California, USA).

In this study, we aimed to establish the relative effectiveness and safety of intravitreal bevacizumab (IVB) as compared to laser photocoagulation in APROP.

7.2 Method

We analyzed retrospectively all the files of the consecutive infants with APROP that we treated either by laser photocoagulation or with IVB between January 1, 2006 and December 31, 2013 and were followed for at least 60 weeks (for the laser group) and 80 weeks (for the IVB group). The overall follow-up ranged between 60 and 144 weeks from the treatment. The study was in agreement with the declaration of Helsinki (1964), and it has the approval of the ethics committee of our university.

Main outcome measures are represented by APROP regression, and the structural outcome associated either with laser photocoagulation or with IVB.

7.2.1 Medical intervention

In APROP we perform treatment (laser or IVB) within 24 hours from diagnosis. Before the intervention, a mixture of tropicamide 0.5% and phenylephrine 2.5% was instilled four times, every 15 minutes in order to obtain pupil dilatation. All laser treatments were performed under analgesia and sedation in the neonatology unit. Laser energy was delivered transpupillary from a portable diode laser having the emission of 810 nm, through the indirect ophthalmoscope. The lids were maintained open with a lid speculum, and the light and laser energy were focalized on the retina with the help of a + 28 diopters lens. We started laser photocoagulation of the retina with a power of 150 mW which we increased gradually up to the obtaining of the desired effect (whitish burn on the retina). We did not exceed 300 mW, the exposure time was 200 ms, and the spot dimension was 200 microns in all circumstances. We applied between 4000 and

6000 burns per eye in 1 or 2 sessions, according to the amount of the nonvascularized retina. The first postlaser checkup took place at 6–7 days and continued every 6–7 days, until there was evidence of APROP regression. If APROP failed to regress, re-treatment was carried out immediately. The frequency of checkups was determined by the clinical course of the disease.

We injected bevacizumab intravitreally for APROP according to the following guidelines: topical anesthesia with 0.5% proparacaine hydrochloride administered three times, every 2 minutes, topical administration of betadine 5%, fixation of the lid speculum, and injection of 0.025 ml (0.625 mg) bevacizumab at 1.5–1.75 mm from the limbus (in the pars plicata), with a 30G needle, perpendicularly on the globe, aiming the center of the eyeball. For the next 3 days, topical tobramycin eye drops were instilled five times/day. The first checkup took place the next day (for the risk of endophthalmitis) and then 7 days following the injection. The follow-up continued every week and then according to the clinical course of the disease.

7.2.2 Follow-up

The infants treated by laser were followed for at least 60 weeks, every month, whereas the ones treated with IVB were followed for at least 80 weeks, every 2 weeks for the first 3 months and then every month. The follow-up was discontinued when full vascularization of the retina was noticed. The exams were performed by three ophthalmologists trained in ROP. In the same time, the patients were followed by pediatricians for the risk of systemic complications related to intravitreal anti-VEGF therapy.

7.2.3 Anatomical outcome

The anatomical outcome was evaluated by indirect ophthalmoscopy. The following signs were considered positive outcome: good pupil dilation and the decrease/disappearance of retinal vessel tortuosity and of the neovascularization. In the IVB group, normal development of the retinal vessels toward periphery was noted. The aggravation of APROP was defined if "plus disease" and/or neovascularization persisted/reappeared, and there were signs of retinal detachment. In these circumstances, laser photocoagulation was added if possible.

7.2.4 Statistical analysis

Statistical analysis was performed using Microsoft Excel and IBM SPSS (version 23.0).

7.3 Results

Between January 1, 2006 and December 31, 2013, we treated 23 infants with APROP. The laser group includes 6 APROP infants and the intravitreal bevacizumab (IVB group) and 17 APROP infants. In both groups, the treatment was bilateral.

7.3.1 Evolution following treatment

APROP treated by laser totalized 24 eyes and by bevacizumab, 34 eyes. Among the laser-treated eyes, the outcome was favorable in 18 eyes (75%), and within the IVB-treated eyes, result was favorable in 29 eyes (85.29%). Chi-square test and Fisher exact test prove no statistically significant difference: p = 0.419 and p = 0.412, respectively.

We needed to repeat laser treatment in 10 of the 24 eyes with APROP (41.66%) with good outcome in 8 of them. Supplementary laser spots were applied on the skipped areas toward the macula.

APROP regressed in 29 eyes (85.29%) from the IVB-treated group and failed to regress in five eyes (14.71%). In three of the five eyes, laser photocoagulation was carried out, with favorable outcome in all of them. In the remaining two eyes, laser treatment could not be performed due to the lack of visualization.

7.3.2 Comparative evolution after treatment between the two groups

The observed differences between the two groups are statistically significant, as proved by McNemar's test (p < 0.001). Global success rate (bilateral or unilateral regression) versus unsuccessful treatment was higher for IVB (94, 12% of cases) against laser photocoagulation (66, 66%), but no statistically significance higher (Chi-square test p = 0.420, Fisher exact test p = 0.462).

After excluding the infants with bad outcome, who came from the same NICU, the difference between the two groups regarding regression rate is no longer significant: 85.29% in the IVB group and 81.25% in the laser photocoagulation group (p > 0.05).

Treatment worked quicker within the IVB group, as compared to the laser photocoagulation group.

The bad outcome was identified 1 week after treatment, in all the 16 eyes within this series (11 from the laser photocoagulation group and 5 from the IVB group). We had no late recurrence in this series.

7.4 Discussion

7.4.1 Indirect diode laser photocoagulation for APROP

Laser photocoagulation of the retina is the gold standard in the treatment of ROP, and it proved its efficacy in more than 90% of ROP cases [18]. On the other hand, laser destroys the retina, and complications were cited in relation to it: cornea, iris and lens burns, hyphema, uveitis, retinal hemorrhages, and choroidal ruptures [19]. In our series, we report two cases of mild anterior uveitis following laser photocoagulation for APROP, with prompt resolution following mydriatic and anti-inflammatory eye drops.

Laser photocoagulation does not address the underlying cause of the disease [18]. Zone 1 APROP is known to have worse prognosis following laser photocoagulation, as compared to the classical form of the disease [20].

Because of the lack of landmarks in APROP, laser photocoagulation of the retina toward the posterior pole is difficult, and sometimes untreated areas of the avascular retina remain as a source of VEGF explaining the progression of the disease. By consequence, one single session of laser treatment is often insufficient in APROP.

Within the laser photocoagulation group, APROP final failure rate was 45.83%, represented by 11 eyes from 7 infants (four, bilaterally and three, unilaterally). From these seven cases, five came from the same neonatal unit and totalize eight eyes with bad outcome (three, bilaterally and two, unilaterally). This observation can lead us to the supposition that the inadequate neonatal care and oxygen administration might be at the origin of the severity and unresponsiveness to the laser treatment in these cases.

If we exclude these eight eyes from our analysis, the success rate following laser photocoagulation for APROP becomes 81.25% (in 13 of the remaining 16 cases, APROP could be stopped by laser treatment).

7.4.2 IVB for APROP in our series

APROP regression rate following IVB was 85.29% in our series (29 of the 34 eyes). We added laser photocoagulation in all the five eyes with lack of regression following IVB, with good outcome in three of them. The two eyes with final poor outcome belonged to different infants.

We did not identify any local complication subsequent to IVB in our group. No late reactivation of the disease was present.

7.4.3 IVB versus laser photocoagulation in the treatment of APROP

The main reason that determined us to replace laser photocoagulation with IVB in APROP was the high failure rate in this form of ROP, following laser treatment, in our practice, which is in agreement with data in the literature (45.83%) [21]. Besides, there are other disadvantages of laser treatment for APROP: the need to apply many laser spots during long and laborious sessions and the need to repeat laser because often at the moment of treatment there are no well-defined landmarks between the vascularized and the nonvascularized retina (typical feature of APROP). Often pupils do not dilate well in these severe cases, and vitreous hemorrhage can be associated, making laser treatment inadequate. The general status of the infant is often severe in APROP cases, making laser treatment risky for the patient's life. Finally, IVB does not destroy the retina as opposed to laser which ablates the nonvascularized retina in order to keep alive its vascular part. [21].

APROP regression rate was significantly better following IVB as compared with laser photocoagulation in our series. However, when we remove from the laser photocoagulation group, the infants with bad outcome, who came from the same NICU, the difference is no longer significant.

Another major advantage of IVB over laser is the continuation of retinal vascularization following treatment up to the periphery [20]. This observation was verified in our series. Anti-VEGF and laser act by different mechanisms in stopping the progression of ROP toward retinal detachment. Whereas laser photocoagulation destroys the source of VEGF (ischemic retina), anti-VEGF annihilates also the VEGF already present in the vitreous. This explains the quicker response and higher efficacy of IVB as compared to laser in APROP.

According to our experience, all bad outcomes were identified 1 week after treatment. Therefore, we consider them as unresponsiveness to treatment, not late recurrences [21].

7.4.4 Asymmetric response to treatment

We identified asymmetric response to treatment in six cases: three from the laser group and three from the IVB group. The possible explanation of this outcome might be the unequal development of the eyes which also explains the rare situation of unilateral ROP.

7.4.5 Safety issues related to anti-VEGF therapy

The main issue related to IVB treatment is its safety. There is proof that following IVB injections the serum VEGF levels decrease and anti-VEGF was found in the systemic circulation [21]. It is known that in ROP the blood-retinal barrier is broken down, allowing the exit of anti-VEGF in the systemic circulation, while the infant is still during the process of organogenesis. Concern comes from the fact that VEGF is necessary for the development of the lungs, brain, kidneys, and skeleton. VEGF also acts as a neural survivor factor inside the eye, and its suppression might prevent the development of neural components in the retina [21].

7.4.6 Comparison between laser and IVB in the treatment of ROP

The advantages of IVB over laser photocoagulation in the treatment of ROP are related to its simplicity; short duration; lack of retinal destruction, conducting under topical anesthesia; lower price; and possibility to be performed in the eyes with small pupils and hazy media and in infants with poor general condition in which laser treatment under general anesthesia would be risky [21]. As proved by our series, IVB allows further development of retinal normal vascularization up to periphery, as opposed to laser. However, IVB is not risk free as far as local complications are considered. Lens injury, intraocular hemorrhage, retinal detachment, and endophthalmitis are possible, but they were not reported in the literature so far.

According to our experience, the most important advantage of IVB as compared to laser treatment is the better outcome in APROP, as published by other authors [21]. In this context, IVB represents our first therapeutic indication for APROP, even if the systemic safety issues were not fully addressed [21].

In a study that compared laser with bevacizumab in ROP and published in 2015, similar results were reported in the two groups, but it included all ROP cases, not just the severe ones (APROP) [22].

Other authors found higher recurrence rate of ROP following IVB as compared to laser, but within the laser group, macular ectopia had a higher incidence [23]. This observation is in agreement with our study that identified macular ectopia only in one case from the laser treated group.

In a previously published study, we showed that in the IVB-treated eyes, the retinal vascularization continued up to the periphery, unlike with laser [24].

Another observation of this comparative study is that the response to IVB was quicker than following laser. The explanation is represented by the fact that anti-VEGF suppresses not only the VEGF in the retina (such as laser does) but also the VEGF which is already released in the vitreous.

8. Conclusion

8.1 Personal experience

Intravitreal bevacizumab has emerged as a very useful tool in the treatment of ROP. We found a statistically significant higher APROP regression rate after IVB, as compared to laser photocoagulation in our series. IVB is much shorter, easier, accessible, and less expensive than laser photocoagulation. We could perform IVB in the eyes with small pupils and hazy media. By consequence, bevacizumab given intravitreally replaced laser in APROP, becoming the standard of care in this severe form of ROP, in our practice.

8.2 General

Progress in neonatal care was associated with higher survival rates of low birth weight and low gestational age newborns.

ROP is a biphasic disease: the first phase (from the moment of birth to 31–32 weeks postconceptional age) is called hyperoxic and it leads to the arrest of the normal retinal development, and the second phase (from 32- to 36-week postconceptional age) is called hypoxic with overexpression of VEGF, IGF-1, and oxidative damage with subsequent new vessel growth and retinal detachment.

The Early Treatment for ROP study (ETROP) reclassified ROP according to the required attitude: type 1, ROP requiring treatment and type 2, ROP requiring closely monitoring. APROP is a very severe type 1 ROP characterized by rapid evolution toward retinal detachment if not addressed accordingly.

ROP screening should be made by trained ophthalmologists and started at 4–6 weeks after birth or at PCA 31 weeks whichever is later and continued up to the complete vascularization of the retina.

The most important factor to prevent ROP is preventing premature birth.

The gold standard for the treatment of ROP is indirect laser photocoagulation of the nonvascularized retina. Clinical studies conducted during the last years proved the superior efficacy of IVB over laser in APROP as well as its other advantages.

Research in the field of angiogenesis led to a number of new ways to prevent ROP progression: targeting the insulin growth factor (IGF-1) pathway and dietary supplementation with omega-3 polyunsaturated fatty acids (PUFA).

Acknowledgements

This study was funded by grant number PED 156, Executive Agency for Higher Education, Research, Development, and Innovation Funding, Romania.

Conflict of interest

The author declares no conflict of interest related to the publication of this chapter.

Author details

Simona Delia Nicoară
Department of Ophthalmology, "Iuliu Hațieganu" University of Medicine and Pharmacy, Cluj-Napoca, Romania

*Address all correspondence to: simonanicoara1@gmail.com

IntechOpen

References

[1] Good WV, Carden SM. Retinopathy of prematurity. British Journal of Ophthalmology. 2006;**90**(3):254-255. DOI: 10.1136/bjo.2005.081166

[2] Salgado CM, Celik Y, Vanderveen DK. Anterior segment complications after diode laser photocoagulation for prethreshold retinopathy of prematurity. American Journal of Ophthalmology. 2010;**150**(1):6-9. DOI: 10.1016/j.ajo.2009.12.017

[3] Wilkinson AR, Haines L, Head K, Fielder AR. UK retinopathy of prematurity guideline. Early Human Development. 2008;**84**(2):71-74. DOI: 10.1016/j.earlhumdev.2007.12.004

[4] Jalali S, Matalia J, Hussain A, Anand R. Modification of screening criteria for retinopathy of prematurity in India and other middle-income countries. American Journal of Ophthalmology. 2006;**141**(5):966-968. DOI: 10.1016/j.ajo.2005.12.016

[5] Gilbert C, Rahi J, Eckstein M, O'Sullivan J, Foster A. Retinopathy of prematurity in middle-income countries. Lancet. 1997;**350**(9070):12-14. DOI: 10.1016/S0140-6736(97)01107-0

[6] Suelves AM, Shulman JP. Current screening and treatments in retinopathy of prematurity in the US. Eye and Brain. 2016;**8**(1):37-43. DOI: 10.2147/EB.S94439

[7] International Committee for the Classification of Retinopathy of Prematurity. The International Classification of Retinopathy of Prematurity revisited. Archives of Ophthalmology. 2005;**123**(7):991-999. DOI: 10.1001/archopht.123.7.991

[8] Cryotherapy for Retinopathy of Prematurity Cooperative Group. Multicenter trial of cryotherapy for retinopathy of prematurity: Preliminary results. Archives of Ophthalmology. 1988;**106**(4):471-479. DOI: 10.1001/archopht.1988.01060130517027

[9] Kieselbach GF, Ramharter A, Baldissera I, Kralinger MT. Laser photocoagulation for retinopathy of prematurity: Structural and functional outcome. Acta Ophthalmologica Scandinavica. 2006;**84**(1):21-26. DOI: 10.1111/j.1600-0420.2005.00548.x

[10] Jing C, Stahl A, Hellstrom A, Smith LS. Current update on retinopathy of prematurity: Screening and treatment. Current Opinion in Pediatrics. 2011;**23**(2):173-178. DOI: 10.1097/mop.0b013e3283423f35

[11] Sato T, Kusaka S, Shimojo H, Fujikado T. Simultaneous analyses of vitreous levels of 27 cytokines in eyes with retinopathy of prematurity. Ophthalmology. 2009;**116**(11):2165-2169. DOI: 10.1016/j.ophtha.2009.04.026

[12] Sonmez K, Drenser KA, Capone A Jr, Trese MT. Vitreous levels of stromal cell-derived factor 1 and vascular endothelial growth factor in patients with retinopathy of prematurity. Ophthalmology. 2008;**115**(6):1065-1070. DOI: 10.1016/j.ophtha.2007.08.050

[13] Sato T, Kusaka S, Shimojo H, Fujikado T. Vitreous levels of erythropoietin and vascular endothelial growth factor in eyes with retinopathy of prematurity. Ophthalmology. 2009;**116**(9):1599-1603. DOI: 10.1016/j.ophtha.2008.12.023

[14] Aiello LP, Pierce EA, Foley ED, et al. Suppression of retinal neovascularization in vivo by inhibition of vascular endothelial growth factor (VEGF) using soluble VEGF-receptor chimeric proteins. Proceedings of

the National Academy of Sciences of the United States of America. 1995;**92**(23):10457-10461

[15] Smith LE, Shen W, Perruzzi C, et al. Regulation of vascular endothelial growth factor-dependent retinal neovascularization by insulin-like growth factor-1 receptor. Nature Medicine. 1999;**5**(12):1390-1395. DOI: 10.1038/70963

[16] Shah N, Jadav P, Jean-Baptiste D, Weedon J, Cohen LM, Kim MR. The effect of recombinant human erythropoietin on the development of retinopathy of prematurity. American Journal of Perinatology. 2010;**27**(1):67-71. DOI: 10.1055/s-0029-1224872

[17] Drenser KA, Trese MT, Capone A Jr. Aggressive posterior retinopathy of prematurity. Retina. 2010;**30**(suppl):S37-S40. DOI: 10.1097/IAE.0b013e3181cb6151

[18] Hellström A, Smith LEH, Dammann O. Retinopathy of prematurity. Lancet. 2013;**382**(9902):1445-1457. DOI: 10.1016/S0140-6736(13)60178-6

[19] Laser ROP Study Group. Laser therapy for retinopathy of prematurity. Archives of Ophthalmology. 1994;**112**(2):154-156

[20] Nicoara SD, Nascutzy C, Cristian C, et al. Outcomes and prognostic factors of intravitreal bevacizumab monotherapy in zone I stage 3+ and aggressive posterior retinopathy of prematurity. Journal of Ophthalmology. 2015;**2015**:1-8. DOI: 10.1155/2015/102582

[21] Nicoara SD, Stefanut AC, Nascutzy C, Zaharie G, Toader LE, Drugan T. Regression rates following the treatment of aggressive posterior retinopathy of prematurity with bevacizumab versus laser: 8 year retrospective analysis. Medical Science Monitor. 2016;**22**:1192-1209. DOI: 10.12659/MSM.897095

[22] Maram I, Kamiar M, Nasrin T. Treatment of type 1 retinopathy of prematurity with bevacizumab versus laser. JAAPOS. 2015;**19**:140-144. DOI: 10.12659/MSM.897095

[23] Hwang KC, Hubbard GB, Hutchinson AK, Lambert SR. Outcomes after intravitreal bevacizumab versus laser photocoagulation for retinopathy of prematurity: A 5-year retrospective analysis. Ophthalmology. 2015;**122**:1008-1015. DOI: 10.12659/MSM.897095

[24] Nicoară SD, Nascutzy C, Cristian C, et al. Outcomes and prognostic factors of intravitreal bevacizumab monotherapy in zone I stage 3+ and aggressive posterior retinopathy of prematurity. Journal of Ophthalmology. 2015;**2015**:102582. DOI: 10.1155/2015/102582

Chapter 6

Parent-Carer Education: Reducing the Risks for Neonatal and Infant Mortality

Thillagavathie Pillay

Abstract

In this chapter, the role of engaging parents, family members, partners, significant others and carers (subsequently referred to as parent-carers) as key partners in targeted strategies for reducing the risks associated with neonatal mortality is discussed, especially within the context of less resource-constrained environments. Parent-carer education, sharing information on regionally prevalent risk factors and associations with death in the first 28 days of life and in infancy, can be potentially impactful and could drive behavioural changes, while promoting acquisition of newer life-saving skills such as basic life support training. Such education can be considered participatory learning and action. It affords parent-carers the confidence and knowledge on measures to key risks in infancy, such as the risk of sudden infant death, and how to recognize when their baby may be ill, facilitating timely access to appropriate healthcare services. Potentially, these then empower parent-carers to work with health services proactively in measures to reduce the risks for neonatal mortality.

Keywords: parent-carer education, reducing risks, neonatal mortality

1. Introduction

Neonatal mortality refers to deaths in the first 28 days after birth and contributes to the total burden of mortality in children. Globally, 5.4 million children under 5 years of age died in 2017, of which 2.5 million were neonates [1]. In this millennium alone, there have been overall improvements in survival in children under 5, but the greatest reduction in mortality is seen in those between 1 and 4 years of age. Between 2000 and 2017, there was a 60% worldwide reduction in mortality in this age group. In contrast, neonatal mortality reduced by 41% [1, 2]. Two key factors have influenced this improvement in outcomes: access to healthcare services and maternal education.

A faster rate of decline in childhood mortality rates compared to neonatal death rate results in the latter assuming a higher proportion of the overall burden of deaths in children. This is especially obvious in more developed economies such as in England, where, with relatively lower child and infant death profiles, the proportion of neonatal deaths to those in infancy and childhood is much higher (70%) [3]. As a result, here, the spotlight has now readjusted towards addressing neonatal mortality [4–6]. In this chapter, the potential for further reductions in neonatal mortality is explored, especially in less resource-constrained environments, by focusing on parent-carer education around risks for neonatal mortality, while using learning points from around the world. Potentially, these initiatives empower parent-carers to acquire the necessary skills to manage their baby at risk and also engage in risk-reducing behaviours for the benefit of their baby.

2. Reducing neonatal mortality through parent-carer education

Before embarking on parent education, understanding the risk factors for neonatal mortality is important. In poorly resourced areas, key risk factors and associations are infection, hypothermia, lack of breastfeeding, failure to recognise signs of illness in their baby and failure to provide adequate basic resuscitation at birth. Education packages focused on improving neonatal mortality therefore include information on maintaining warmth; drying; wrapping; skin-to-skin contact; supporting breastfeeding; infection prevention including handwashing, cord care, recognising signs of illness in their newborn baby and infant and basic life support [7].

For neonatal teams in relatively higher resourced environments, where access to public health facilities and general maternal education are less of an issue, and most of the above are routinely adopted, what are other key risk factors and what other kinds of initiatives are needed in order to make a difference to current neonatal mortality rates, and can they work?

In attempting to address this, the key risk factors here for neonatal mortality need to be identified. The most significant of these is prematurity [8–10]. In a report on perinatal mortality from MBRRACE on 2016 deaths, approximately 70% of all extended perinatal deaths occurred preterm, and almost 40% were in less than 28 weeks' gestation [9]. Optimising place of birth for the most vulnerable preterm births less than 26 weeks gestation at birth does reduce their mortality rates [11] and optimising nurse staffing for the care of especially preterm babies in neonatal intensive care units appears to be crucial [12]. Evidence-based or consensus medical and nursing care, robust reviews of mortalities and complex morbidities and sound clinical governance are instinctively important. But, simply improving clinical care provided, and in the correct place, is probably not enough.

By virtue of these babies being born prematurely, much of the potential factors that could influence outcome predate the birth of baby. These include obstetric, maternal health and social factors [13] and are usually out of the bounds of care of neonatal teams. For example, in the risk factors for neonatal mortality in a region in the West Midlands in England, prematurity, being born with low birth weight, congenital abnormalities, born at the extremes of maternal age, late maternal presentation for antenatal care, smoking, not breastfeeding and sudden infant death syndrome (SIDS) were the key associations with infant mortality [8]. All of these are influenced by upstream issues, that is, before birth (except SIDS). Just focusing on care pathways and postnatal care for these babies on neonatal units and in the community will have little impact on their mortality rate. A more multidisciplinary, lateral approach is needed, and there are lessons too, from developments in parent education in resource-limited environments.

Apart from optimising clinical care, what else can *neonatal* teams do? An area of focus for neonatal units could potentially be enhanced primary preventive care [4]. There is evidence that early parental interventions in preterm births are effective in promoting child health [14], and there is possible value in targeting parent-carer empowerment in reducing the risks of mortality for their newly born baby in infancy and beyond. Data on this as a package of care, however, are very limited. Maternal education improves infant, child and maternal mortality globally [15–17]. These relate to mothers' general awareness through education, which empowers women to make better decisions on the care of their baby and themselves. Engaging them in understanding the regional mortality risks for their baby, and their future babies, and what they could do to minimise these where possible may be of value. This kind of awareness of risk factors for infant mortality could provide parents and carers with knowledge that could drive longer term behavioural change that could influence the outcome of current baby, subsequent pregnancies and, in a cascade effect, those of close family members.

A recent project on parent education around the risks of mortality in a region in the West Midlands [8] in England revealed that parental uptake for the education on understanding risks for mortality was well accepted and supported (**Table 1**). Educating parents and carers on the basics of life support, how to manage their choking child and how to recognise that their baby is ill may empower parents and carers, enabling them to initiate preventative intervention earlier, which may be life-saving. Evidence that this can affect short-term behavioural change and empowerment through confidence building in parents appears to be possible [8], but more studies are needed in this regard.

Very informative and should be offered to all parents
I think this should be available to all parents. Found it really useful even after having three babies
All parents should be offered this!
It is a great programme and all parents will benefit from it. I know I have!
Really useful—should be available to all parents
Really appreciate eagerness of staff to come and help us
Include grandparents/relatives; make it compulsory for first-time parents. Make nursing staff more aware for STORK referrals
I can truly say this service has made me feel 100% confident in taking my baby home! Could not be more grateful. Thank you!
Very useful and helpful instructor. Wish all mums had this opportunity.
Really helpful. Get to know things you did not before and understand it better
It is good to help save babies' life. Every parent should do
Very informative, thank you
This made me feel at ease about taking my baby Harry home knowing about the ways to safe sleep. Brilliant today. Thank you very much!
Very good. Helped put my mind at ease should the need arise. Felt very comfortable
Trainer very informative and helpful. Additional advice given on other topics; reassurance given
Covered a lot I wasn't even aware of
Was very useful and has made me aware now as I did not have a clue about any
Absolutely I think all parents should go through this not just ones on neonates unit
Brilliant!!

Table 1.
Selected parent feedback comments for parent/carer training on a neonatal unit in the West Midlands, England. Extracted from [8].

3. The benefits of overall maternal education on infant mortality

The most significant factor globally in reducing mortality for young children under 5 years of age is maternal education, and universal primary education for mothers is an established key focus of the United Nations Millennium Development Goal [17]. Better maternal education decreases not only childhood mortality but also maternal mortality [18] and is evident across resource-constrained and resource-richer environments. This is most striking in the former, where lower levels of maternal education (i.e., less than secondary school education) are significantly associated with neonatal mortality. In resource-richer environments, this effect is less noticeable [19] but prevalent in pockets with lower socio-economic status and lower levels of maternal education [19, 20]. While not easy to tease out, it is assumed that the impact of general maternal education on infant and childhood outcomes relates to empowerment of women to make better decisions over the care of their baby and care of themselves. Therefore, any targeted education, through providing parents and carers with knowledge of risks and associations with neonatal mortality, may contribute to empowering them into making decisions in the best interest of their baby, in an attempt to reduce risks for mortality.

4. Methods of delivering targeted parent-carer education

A synopsis of this can be found in **Table 2**.

4.1 One-to-one point-of-care education

This refers to education around a reason for a healthcare visit, usually in the home, or a visiting point. This has its benefits, providing an opportunity for maternal and family engagement with health services and focused learning and behavioural change. It is best reported in resource-constrained environments, as evidenced by the impact of health visits and education on behavioural changes and infant mortality, in women who have recently given birth [21]. Keeping baby warm, dry and wrapped to prevent hypothermia, skin-to-skin contact, breastfeeding and infection prevention, including delivering in a clean environment, handwashing, cord care and knowing what the signs of illness are in their baby, are key aspects of shared knowledge [21]. Guidelines for postnatal care of the mother and newborn, especially in resource-limited environments, were produced by the World Health Organisation ([22], **Table 3**), and these include parent education via home visits in the first week after birth and at least three additional postnatal contact points in the first 6 weeks of life.

In resource-richer environments, for example, England, similar 1:1 point-of-care visits at home usually occur post-delivery, initially by midwives and later by healthcare workers. NICE Guidelines on 1:1 postnatal care [23] guide the basic requirements for routine postnatal care for women and their babies and their partners and families. Support for feeding, advice on safe sleeping, recognising and dealing with health problems for both mother and baby are included in the quality standard, but there are limitations to its success to date [24]. These are usually delivered by midwives or health visitors, as the primary healthcare contacts for a mother and family with a newly born baby.

Educational engagement with parents and carers on the neonatal unit occurs as per unit policy and can include a wide variety of information supported by online

Method	Example
Home visits by community health care workers [69]	Home visit by community-based worker after birth in India: information shared included breastfeeding, basic care of the baby—temperature control, hygiene, care of the umbilical cord stump, danger signs in the baby and how to use the healthcare system, especially for the sick, or preterm, or low-birth weight baby. There was a significant reduction in neonatal mortality rate in those who received the education [35.7 deaths per 1000 live births compared to those who did not (53.8 per 1000 live births)]
Regular community group sessions by Lady Health Workers [70]	Group sessions by lady health workers in Pakistan included sharing information on immediate newborn care, cord care (cleaning and avoiding the use of traditional materials, such as ash and lead powder), and promotion of exclusive breastfeeding. There was also additional sharing of information on early breastfeeding (within the first hour) use of colostrum, thermoregulation, home care of low-birth weight infants, treatment of neonatal pneumonia, recognising the sick baby and danger signs needing treatment. Here the neonatal mortality rate significantly decreased from 57.3 to 41.3 per 1000 live births.
Community-based package of care in [71]	In India, this package included birth preparedness, clean delivery and cord care, thermal care (including skin-to-skin care), breastfeeding promotion, and danger sign recognition, and in one group a hypothermia indicator. Compared with controls, neonatal mortality rate was significantly reduced by 54%.
Participatory learning and action via women's groups [25]	This was a meta-analysis of seven trials in India, Bangladesh, Nepal, Malawi, estimating the effect of women's group interventions on behavioural outcomes. Women's groups practising PLA showed improved behaviours during and after home deliveries, including the use of safe birthing kits, sterile blade to cut the cord, birth attendant washing hands before delivery, delayed bathing of baby for at least 24 hours and wrapping baby within 10 minutes of birth. Here, neonatal mortality was 32% lower in the clusters that had the intervention.
In resource-richer environments	
Organised support groups	Peer support groups may work on one-to-one or group basis, face-to-face, via telephone, social media or social engagement and include online and physical resources for training and guidance to parents on antenatal, birth and child issues. E.g.: Child birth peer support groups, supporting antenatal, birth and parenting in the UK (NCT); https://www.nct.org.uk/ E.g.: BLISS charity for sick and preterm babies; https://www.bliss.org.uk/
Support groups: local, regional, national and international [72]	E.g.: Breastfeeding support may be delivered on one-to-one or group format, at the bedside while in hospital and in the home. Breastfeeding support workers, nurses and breastfeeding buddies may be local and regional and hospital or community based. There also exists international organisational support through La Leche League International; https://www.llli.org/
Support for specialised conditions/ congenital anomalies	These are usually groups based on national or international need and include for example the national Down syndrome group in the UK, and its international counterpart—Down syndrome international, which co-ordinates working with and advocating the case for children with Down syndrome in over 136 countries around the world.

Table 2.
Examples of parent-carer engagement: examples from around the world.

1: Timing of discharge from a health facility after birth	After an uncomplicated vaginal birth in a health facility, healthy mothers and babies should receive care in the facility for at least 24 hours after birth.
2: Number and timing of postnatal contacts	If birth is at home, the first postnatal contact should be as early as possible within 24 hours of birth. At least three additional postnatal contacts are recommended for all mothers and babies, on day 3, between days 7 and 14 after birth, and 6 weeks after birth.
3: Home visits for postnatal care	If birth is in a health facility, mothers and babies should receive postnatal care in the facility for at least 24 hours after birth. Home visits in the first week after birth are recommended for care of the mother and her baby.
4: Assessment of the baby	The following signs should be assessed during each postnatal care contact and the baby should be referred for further evaluation if any of the signs is present: *stopped feeding well, history of convulsions, fast breathing (breathing rate 60 per minute), severe chest in-drawing, no spontaneous movement, fever (temperature 37.5°C), low body temperature (temperature < 35.5°C), any jaundice in first 24 hours of life, or yellow palms and soles at any age.* The family should be encouraged to seek health care early if they identify any of the above danger signs in between postnatal care visits.
5: Exclusive breastfeeding	All babies should be exclusively breastfed from birth until 6 months of age. Mothers should be counselled and provided support for exclusive breastfeeding at each postnatal contact.
6: Cord care	Daily chlorhexidine application to the umbilical cord stump during the first week of life is recommended for babies who are born at home in settings with high neonatal mortality (30 or more neonatal deaths per 1000 live births). Clean, dry cord care is recommended for babies born in health facilities and at home in low neonatal mortality settings. Use of chlorhexidine in these situations may be considered only to replace application of a harmful traditional substance to the cord stump.
7: Other postnatal care	Bathing should be delayed until 24 hours after birth. If this is not possible, bathing should be delayed for at least 6 hours. Appropriate clothing of the baby for ambient temperature is recommended. This means one to two layers of clothes more than adults, and use of hats/caps. The mother and baby should not be separated and should stay in the same room 24 hours a day. Communication and play with the baby should be encouraged. Immunisation should be promoted as per existing WHO guidelines. Preterm and low-birth weight babies should be identified immediately after birth and should be provided special care as per existing WHO guidelines.

Table 3.
WHO recommendation on postnatal care for newborn babies, 2013 [22].

resources and paper reading material. Guidance on basic life support is offered by some, but specific packages of information targeting knowledge around key risk factors on neonatal mortality are usually not presented in such a format to parents and carers. These may, however, be a useful point-of-care opportunity for education and training [8].

4.2 Centre-based peer group education

Participatory learning and action programmes promoted by the World Health Organization drive behavioural change through parent and community engagement [25].

Support groups work through community engagement, in which mothers develop and implement their own strategies for improvement, through shared peer group learning with a facilitator. The women are empowered to make improvements for their own communities, which result in behavioural changes that were more effective than simple traditional teacher/student model. In a trial in India, neonatal mortality reduced by 45%, with behavioural changes towards better hygiene practices and better newborn care, such as cord care, delivering in a clean environment and early breastfeeding [26].

In higher resourced environments, participatory learning and action can apply as well, with parents being offered information on risks for neonatal and infant mortality, knowledge on basic life support and choking, reducing the risks for sudden infant death and promoting safe sleeping and recognising signs of illness in their infant [8].

4.3 Local, regional and national support groups

In resource-richer environments, peer groups supporting the new mother may be driven by health care or by the community. Mother and baby peer groups or new parent groups are a useful way of engaging parents and family members [27] and can be local, regional or national such as BLISS, which is a national charity for sick and premature babies [28] in England. These may be one-to-one engagements or group interaction depending on resources and availability and include online resources for learning and communicating. Examples of these are shown in **Table 2**.

The benefits of these kinds of educational thrust on reducing mortality may be less obvious where health care is equitable to all [19], but still of value as such environments do have pockets of poorer educational levels [20], linked with greater mortality. It may be appropriate to extrapolate that the benefits of maternal peer and group education in contributing to behavioural changes that reduce the risk of mortality can possibly also apply to resource-richer environments. In the USA, an Advisory Committee on Infant Mortality identified the value of a multimedia approach in the preventive campaign needed to reduce infant mortality [29]. They suggest a life course perspective on infant mortality reduction, urging an approach that includes health promotion and optimisation throughout the course of life, in a clinical and population-based manner. Such a perspective should include focused parent-carer education and empowerment through education on risks for infant mortality. This could mean that parents have a better idea of how best and when to seek help for their baby who may be getting ill, that is, early initiation of preventative care. Although widely prevalent in higher resourced economies, very little has been studied in this regard, and this is being mapped better in more resource-constrained settings [30].

5. What should a parent-carer education package aimed at reducing the risks for infant mortality comprise?

Key parameters are driven by local epidemiological needs. It is likely that even in areas that do adopt a primary prevention package the contents will change depending on societal needs. In resource-limited environments with poor access to health care, basic hygiene around delivery, cord care, keeping baby dry, wrapped and warm, immunizations, basic life support and breastfeeding may be key [21, 22]. In less resource-constrained environments, where most of the above are standard practice, other areas may be relevant. In the sections below, some of these are described.

5.1 Breastfeeding education and infant mortality

The benefits of breastfeeding on reducing infant mortality and morbidity are widely accepted. In 2003, the Lancet published data [31] that of all children who died under the age of 5 years, 12% of these deaths could have been prevented if they were effectively breastfed as infants. This amounted to roughly 800,000 lives in low- and middle-income countries per year. In their systematic review, Sankar et al. [32] showed that the relative risk for all-cause mortality in infants under 6 months of age and not breastfed was 14.4, 4.8 in those partially breastfed and 1.5 in those completely breastfed. For children 6–23 months of age, they demonstrated up to a two-fold higher mortality (RR 1.97 [1.45–2.67]) if not breastfed, when compared to those who were. Exclusive breastfeeds are also associated with lower mortality and infection rates [33], and this impact can be seen as early as with breastfeeds given within the first hour of life [34–36]. Maternal awareness, education and support for breastfeeding to improve breastfeeding rates are therefore a critical part of the parent empowerment, in reducing infant mortality.

These benefits exist in all resource settings. For example, in Washington, Alaska, Maine, Nebraska and Ohio, promotion of the Baby Friendly Hospital Initiative saw benefits of this for mothers of lower education which were significant, increasing the breastfeeding rates for >4 weeks of life here (p = 0.02) [37]. These provide evidence for the continued thrust for promoting breastfeeding as a potential protective factor against the risk of neonatal and infant mortality, even in resource-richer environments. The Baby Friendly Initiative, developed by UNICEF, promotes breastfeeding as part of its thrust to support families with feeding, enabling the development of close relationships for the best start in life for babies.

5.2 Smoking cessation and infant mortality

The negative effects of prenatal, natal and postnatal smoking on morbidity and mortality in infants are widely described [38, 39] and include premature births, low-birth weight babies which are themselves at risk for mortality and an increased risk for sudden infant death. Smoking cessation in pregnancy or prenatally, or even postnatally, is complex. Risk factors for smoking include having a smoking partner, with a lower risk where there is higher maternal education level [40]. Mass campaigns can potentially influence smoking cessation rates in pregnancy [41]. In three states in the USA, those smokers exposed to a CDC smoking cessation campaign in pregnancy had a reduction in smoking by the third trimester compared to those who were not exposed to the campaign (34.7 vs. 32.9%; p < 0.001). In a systematic review and meta-analysis of 54 studies encompassing 55,584 women who smoked before their pregnancy, Riaz et al. [42] noted that higher educational level, higher socio-economic status, low exposure to second-hand smoke and planned breastfeeding were associated with cessation of smoking during pregnancy. So, there is potential value, extrapolating from these that an awareness programme could influence smoking cessation rates in association with pregnancy/after birth, targeting not only mothers, but their partners, significant others and family members.

Education versus incentive-based systems to reduce smoking may work to different degrees. These modern alternatives to conventional educational and awareness campaigns could include mobile apps, ipad programmes and text messages [43, 44]. But simply offering education may not be adequate, and there is much more to be done to understand this. Barriers to smoking cessation are multi-fold and may exceed support pathways. In an NIHR HTA assessment of these [45], partners' support, willingness to change smoking behaviour and the smoking dynamics within relationships mattered, and delivery of information is a key barrier than can potentially be overcome with the appropriate educational drives. At the same time, it is important to note that up to 50% of women who stop smoking during their pregnancy resume within 6 months after birth [46]. There may be a hard core of individual mothers/parents who are unable to stop smoking, even knowing the risks to their baby. Some evidence exists that specific behavioural techniques may have an impact on prenatal smoking cessation [47–49], but the complexities around cessation in relation to pregnancy and childbirth need further interventional analysis. Despite these limitations, there may still be the benefit of incorporating smoking cessation information into parent awareness packages [8], while awaiting more effective interventions and primary preventive packages.

5.3 Safe sleep

Safe sleep programmes can make a difference to the risks of sudden infant death syndrome. In parts of the USA, interventions such as these halved the rate of infant deaths from 1.08/1000 to 0.48/1000. Research suggests that education of caregivers does result in improved understanding of behaviours that promote safe sleep and reduce the risk of SIDS [50]. Simple measures such as position of sleeping have changed SIDS rates dramatically [51]. And parent and carer education is a key directive for future reductions in this area [52]. Evidence that discharge from hospital programmes do make a difference is also emerging [53] in a pilot trial of promoting safe sleep patterns in mothers of preterm babies, who have a doubled risk of SIDS; and there is also acknowledgement that this group especially should be targeted for educational interventions to reduce the risk of SIDS. Simple educational campaigns en masse may not have the desired effect [54, 55] and additional measures may be needed such as 1:1 educational drives. These can comfortably be delivered in 1:1 or peer group packages supported by neonatal units, midwives and health care visitors as part of the point-of-care programme of education for parents and carers.

5.4 Basic life support training

Basic life support at birth is critical, and a standard practice in higher income settings where healthcare support exists at the time of birth. However, even for home births and births outside of healthcare facilities, this skill is essential. In their review on neonatal resuscitation in low-income settings, Wall et al. [56] noted that the major burden of resuscitation at birth (approximately 10 million babies do not breathe at birth, of which 6 million require basic life support) is in low-income settings. Here, they suggest that local education of community health workers can make a difference to the rate of deaths at the time of birth (termed intrapartum deaths).

In higher income settings, where there are healthcare workers trained in basic life support, there still exists a need for parent-carer education and awareness. Acute life-threatening events in infancy are the next area of concern and can affect babies as young as 0–3 months of age [57]. Bystander CPR with and without dispatcher instructions improved 1-month neurological outcomes favourably (adjusted OR 1.81 and 1.68) when compared to no bystander CPR in children with out-of-hospital cardiac arrests [58], and survival after shockable arrests was higher when delivered by a first responder or public AED rather than a paramedic (83.3 vs. 40% p = 0.04) [59]. In reporting on the Committee on Pediatric Emergency Medicine in the USA, Callahan and colleagues advocate that paediatricians should encourage training of basic life support to parents, children, caregivers, school personnel and lay members of the public [60]. Many neonatal units do offer basic life support training for parents and carers when their baby is due to leave their unit; these boost parent confidence in being able to cope with their infant after discharge from hospital.

5.5 Kangaroo care and infant mortality

Skin-to-skin contact via Kangaroo care [61] is also an important part of a care package especially for preterm births. When compared to conventional care, Kangaroo mother care was associated with 36% lower mortality (RR 0.64), a lower risk of neonatal sepsis (RR 0.53), hypothermia (RR 0.22), hypoglycaemia (RR 0.12), hospital readmission (RR 0.42) and increased rate of exclusive breastfeeding (RR 1.50; 95% CI 1.26, 1.78) [62]. Educating and empowering mothers, on the value of such care packages, is important in reducing morbidities especially in low-birth weight infants.

5.6 Reducing the risks for congenital abnormalities

Congenital abnormalities are a major cause of infant mortality in higher resource environments, with variation between ethnic groups and a strong association with consanguinity [63, 64]. Reducing the risks for life-threatening congenital abnormalities [65] (either through the condition itself, or through its association with preterm birth) is dependent on parental awareness regarding the risks of congenital abnormality pre-conceptually, availability and uptake of screening for major congenital abnormalities, the potential for intervention, and parent perspectives on termination of pregnancy, should they carry a baby with a lethal/potentially lethal condition in utero. Where possible, parent education to raise awareness regarding the likelihood of a congenital abnormality should be discussed in the context of consanguinity and the elderly mother.

5.7 Reducing the risk of preterm birth

Risk factors for preterm birth include, among a wide array of clinical scenarios, poor maternal health, maternal infections, smoking and alcohol use in pregnancy, multiple births and extremes of maternal age [66]. The World Health Organisation [67] has set out basic advice to reduce preterm births and these include promoting a healthy pregnancy by supporting: (a) a healthy diet, (b) optimal nutrition, (c) advice on tobacco use in pregnancy, (d) advice on alcohol use in pregnancy, (e) antenatal support and scanning to detect gestational age and multiple births, (f) better access to contraceptives, (g) management of risk factors such as infections and (h) increased maternal empowerment.

In higher resource settings, strategies for prevention of preterm births include: (a) prevention of non-medically indicated late preterm/early term births, (b) progesterone supplementation, (c) cervical cerclage, (d) tobacco control and prevention of smoking in pregnancy, (e) judicious use of fertility treatments and (f) dedicated preterm birth prevention clinics [68].

All of these aspects relate to upstream events prior to birth of the baby, but still hold benefit in parent-carer education, for the ripple effect that it may have on communities, and also for guiding care around the subsequent pregnancy.

6. Conclusion

Parent education programmes, targeted around understanding and, thereby, empowering parents with knowledge around the risks of neonatal and infant mortality, are an intuitively important adjunct to neonatal clinical care. Its role in preventive neonatal care may be strong, for its potential benefits on behavioural changes that enable reduced risks for the current and subsequent pregnancies. Getting parents actively engaged in programmes that work *with* them for the betterment of their baby, their subsequent babies and their communities may be the key to change for the future. This embraces patient and public (i.e., parents/family members/significant others and carers) involvement in taking ownership of, and making a greater contribution to their overall health, and to that of their families.

What is now needed are focused thrusts around parent education and empowerment, based on local risk factors and associations with neonatal mortality, combined with robust scientific research to assess the impact, if any, of such programmes.

Acknowledgements

To the Royal Wolverhampton NHS Trust, its Neonatal Unit, parents and babies who participated, Wolverhampton Public Health and to its commissioning group for supporting this programme.

Conflict of interest

There is no conflict of interest.

Author details

Thillagavathie Pillay[1,2*]

1 School of Medicine and Clinical Practice, Faculty of Science and Engineering, University of Wolverhampton, Royal Wolverhampton NHS Trust, Wolverhampton, United Kingdom

2 Department of Health Sciences, College of Life Sciences, University of Leicester, Leicester, United Kingdom

*Address all correspondence to: tilly.pillay@nhs.net

IntechOpen

References

[1] United Nations Inter-agency group for Child Mortality Estimation. Levels and Trends in Child Mortality. Report 2018. Available from: http://childmorta lity.org/files_v22/download/UN% 20IGME%20Child%20Mortality%20Re port%202018.pdf [Accessed 15-10-2018]

[2] United Nations Inter-agency Group for Child Mortality. Estimation (UN IGME), Levels & Trends in Child Mortality: Report 2017. Estimates Developed by the UN Inter-agency Group for Child Mortality Estimation', United Nations Children's Fund, New York. 2017

[3] Public Health England. Facts and Figures on Infant Mortality and Stillbirths. National Child and Maternal Health Intelligence Network, 2014. Available from: http://webarchive.na tionalarchives.gov.uk/20170302101718/ http://www.chimat.org.uk/maternity/ factsandfigures [Date Accessed: 22-08-2018]

[4] Pillay T. Parent, family and carer empowerment and neonatal mortality: Stretching the boundaries for neonatal units. Journal of Neonatal Nursing. 2018;4:289-290. DOI: 10.1016/j. jnn.2018.07.006

[5] Public Health England. Mortality. Infant Mortality and Stillbirths Profile. Available from: https://fingertips.phe. org.uk/profile-group/child-health/prof ile/child-health-mortality [Date Accessed: 22-08-2018]

[6] MBRRACE-UK: Mothers and Babies: Reducing Risk through Audits and Confidential Enquiries across the UK. https://www.npeu.ox.ac.uk/mbrrace-uk [Accessed: 15-10-2018]

[7] Enweronu-Laryea C, Dickson KE, Moxon SG, et al. Basic newborn care and neonatal resuscitation: A multi-country analysis of health system bottlenecks and potential solutions. BMC Pregnancy and Childbirth. 2015;15 (Supp. 2):S4

[8] Pillay T, Porter K, Marson S. Developing an early life parent education programme in response to high infant mortality rates. Journal of Neonatal Nursing. 2017;23(5):242-243

[9] MBRRACE Perinatal Mortality Surveillance Report. UK Perinatal Deaths for Births from January to December 2016. Summary Report. Available from: https://www.npeu.ox. ac.uk/downloads/files/mbrrace-uk/ reports/MBRRACE-UK%20Perinatal% 20Surveillance%20Summary%20Report %20for%202016%20-%20June% 202018.pdf [Date Accessed: 23-08-2018]

[10] Institute of Medicine (US) Committee on Understanding Premature Birth and Assuring Healthy Outcomes. In: Behrman RE, Butler AS, editors. Preterm Birth: Causes, Consequences, and Prevention. Washington (DC): National Academies Press (US); 2007. 10, Mortality and Acute Complications in Preterm Infants. Available from: https://www.ncbi.nlm. nih.gov/books/NBK11385/

[11] Marlow N, Bennett C, Draper ES, Hennessy EM, Morgan AS, Costeloe KL. Perinatal outcomes for extremely preterm babies in relation to place of birth in England: The EPICure 2 study. Archives of Disease in Childhood. Fetal and Neonatal Edition. 2014;99(3):F181-F188. DOI: 10.1136/archdischild-2013-305555

[12] Watson SI, Arulampalam W, Petrou S, et al. The effects of a one-to-one nurse-to-patient ratio on the mortality rate in neonatal intensive care: A retrospective, longitudinal, population-based study.

Archives of Disease in Childhood. Fetal and Neonatal Edition. 2016;**101**(3): F195-F200. DOI: 10.1136/archdischild-2015-309435

[13] Kim D, Saada A. The social determinants of infant mortality and birth outcomes in Western developed nations: A cross-country systematic review. International Journal of Environmental Research and Public Health. 2013;**10**(6):2296-2335. DOI: 10.3390/ijerph10062296

[14] Puthussery S, Chutiyami M, Tseng PC, Kilby L, Kapadia J. Effectiveness of early intervention programs for parents of preterm infants: A meta-review of systematic reviews. Pediatrics. 2016; **137**(1):e20152238. DOI: 10.1542/peds.2015-2238

[15] Sosnaud B. Inequality in infant mortality: Cross-state variation and medical system institutions. Social Problems. 2017. 10.1093/socpro/spx034 [Date Accessed: 23-08-2018]

[16] Cutler DM, Lleras-Muney A. Understanding differences in health behaviors by education. Journal of Health Economics. 2010;**29**(1):1-28. Published online 2009 October. DOI: 10.1016/j.jhealeco.2009.10.003

[17] Veneman AN. Education is key to reducing child mortality: The link between maternal health and education. UN Chronicle. 2007;**XLIV**(4)

[18] Karlsen S, Say L, Souza JP, et al. The relationship between maternal education and mortality among women giving birth in health care institutions: Analysis of the cross sectional WHO Global Survey on Maternal and Perinatal Health. BMC Public Health. 2011;**11**:606

[19] Carlsen F, Grytten J, Eskild A. Maternal education and risk of offspring death; changing patterns from 16 weeks of gestation until one year after birth.

European Journal of Public Health. 2014;**24**(1):157-162

[20] Goldfarb SS, Houser K, Wells BA, Brown Speights JS, Beitsch L, Rust G. Pockets of progress amidst persistent racial disparities in low birthweight rates. PLoS One. 2018;**13**(7):e0201658

[21] Gogia S, Singh Sachdev H. Home visits by community health workers to prevent neonatal deaths in developing countries: A systematic review. Bulletin of the World Health Organization. 2010; **88**:658-666B

[22] World Health Organisation. Recommendations on Post Natal Care of the Mother and Newborn. 2013. Available from: https://www.who.int/maternal_child_adolescent/docume nts/postnatal-care-recommendations/en/ [Accessed: 15-10-2018]

[23] National Institute for Clinical Excellence Quality Standard 37. Post Natal Care. Available from: https://www.nice.org.uk/Guidance/QS37 [Accessed: 15-10-2018]

[24] The Royal College of Midwives. Post Natal Care Planning. Pressure Points. The Case for Better Post Natal Care. Available from: https://www.rcm.org.uk/sites/default/files/Pressure%20Points%20-%20Postnatal%20Care%20Planning%20-%20Web%20Copy.pdf [Accessed: 15-10-2018]

[25] Seward N, Neuman M, Colbourn T, et al. Effects of women's groups practising participatory learning and action on preventive and care-seeking behaviours to reduce neonatal mortality: A meta-analysis of cluster-randomised trials. PLOS Medicine. 2017;**14**(12): e1002467

[26] Tripathy P, Nair N, Barnett S, et al. Effect of a participatory intervention with women's groups on birth outcomes and maternal depression in Jharkhand

and Orissa, India: A cluster-randomised controlled trial. Lancet. 2010;**375**: 1182-1192

[27] Guest EM, Keatinge DR. The value of new parent groups in child and family health nursing. The Journal of Perinatal Education. 2009;**18**(3):12-22. DOI: 10.1624/105812409X461180

[28] BLISS: For Babies Born Sick or Premature. https://www.bliss.org.uk/ [Accessed: 15-10-2018]

[29] Lu MC, Johnson KA. Toward a national strategy on infant mortality. American Journal of Public Health. 2014;**104**(Supp. 1):S13-S16

[30] The International Initiative for Impact Evaluation. Mapping the Evidence on Social, Behavioural and Community Engagement for Reproductive, Maternal, Newborn, Child and Adolescent Health. Available from: http://www.3ieimpact.org/media/filer_public/2017/11/06/3ie_who-rmnch-brief.pdf [Accessed: 22-08-2018]

[31] Jones G, Steketee RW, Black RE, Bhutta ZA, Morris SS. Bellagio child survival study G. How many child deaths can we prevent this year? Lancet. 2003;**362**:65-71

[32] Sankar MJ, Sinha B, Chowdhury R, Bhandari N, Taneja S, Martines J, et al. Optimal breastfeeding practices and infant and child mortality: A systematic review and meta-analysis. Acta Paediatrica. 2015;**104**(467):3-13

[33] Khan J, Vesel L, Bahl R, Martines JC. Timing of breastfeeding initiation and exclusivity of breastfeeding during the first month of life: Effects on neonatal mortality and morbidity–a systematic review and meta-analysis. Maternal and Child Health Journal. 2015;**19**(3): 468-479

[34] Boccolini CS, Carvalho ML, Oliveira MI, Pérez-Escamilla R. Breastfeeding during the first hour of life and neonatal mortality. Jornal de Pediatria. 2013;**89**(2):131-136

[35] Phukan D, Ranjan M, Dwivedi LK. Impact of timing of breastfeeding initiation on neonatal mortality in India. International Breastfeeding Journal. 2018;**13**:27

[36] Smith ER, Chowdhury R, Sinha B, Fawzi W, Edmond KM, Neovita Study Group. Delayed breastfeeding initiation and infant survival: A systematic review and meta-analysis. PLoS One. 2017;**12**(7):e0180722

[37] Hawkins SS, Stern AD, Baum CF, Gillman MW. Evaluating the impact of the Baby-Friendly Hospital Initiative on breast-feeding rates: A multi-state analysis. Public Health Nutrition. 2015;**18**(2):189-197

[38] NHS. Stopping Smoking is the Best Thing You Can do for Your Baby. Available from: https://www.nhs.uk/smokefree/why-quit/smoking-in-pregnancy [Date Accessed: 23-08-2018]

[39] Smoking: Stopping in Pregnancy and after Childbirth. NICE Public Health Guideline 26. Published June 2010. Available from: https://www.nice.org.uk/guidance/ph26/chapter/1-recommendations [Date Accessed: 23-08-2018]

[40] Lamy S, Houivet E, Marret S, Hennart B, et al. Risk factors associated to tobacco and alcohol use in a large French cohort of pregnant women. Archives of Women's Mental Health. 2018. DOI: 10.1007/s00737-018-0892-4. [Epub ahead of print]

[41] England L, Tong VT, Rockhill K, et al. Evaluation of a federally funded mass media campaign and smoking cessation in pregnant women: A population-based study in three states. BMJ Open. 2017;**7**(12):e016826

[42] Riaz M, Lewis S, Naughton F, Ussher M. Predictors of smoking cessation during pregnancy: A systematic review and meta-analysis. Addiction. 2018;**113**(4):610-622

[43] Rathbone AL, Prescott J. The use of mobile apps and SMS messaging as physical and mental health interventions: Systematic review. Journal of Medical Internet Research. 2017;**19**(8):e295

[44] Dotson JAW, Pineda R, Cylkowski H, Amiri S. Development and evaluation of an iPad application to promote knowledge of tobacco use and cessation by pregnant women. Nursing for Women's Health. 2017;**21**(3):174-185

[45] Bauld L, Graham H, Sinclair L, et al. Barriers to and facilitators of smoking cessation in pregnancy and following childbirth: Literature review and qualitative study. Health Technology Assessment. 2017;**21**(36):1-158

[46] Underner M, Pourrat O, Perriot J, Peiffer G, Jaafari N. Smoking cessation and pregnancy. Gynecologie, Obstetrique, Fertilite & Senologie. 2017 Oct;**45**(10):552-557

[47] Wilson SM, Newins AR, Medenblik AM, et al. Contingency Management Versus Psychotherapy for Prenatal Smoking Cessation: A Meta-Analysis of Randomized, Controlled Trials. Womens Health Issues. 2018;**28** pii: S1049-3867(17)30655-2. DOI: 10.1016/j.whi.2018.05.002. [Epub ahead of print]

[48] Wen X, Eiden RD, Justicia-Linde FE, et al. A multicomponent behavioral intervention for smoking cessation during pregnancy: A nonconcurrent multiple-baseline design. Translational Behavioral Medicine. 2018:10. DOI: 10.1093/tbm/iby027

[49] Campbell KA, Fergie L, Coleman-Haynes T, et al. Improving behavioral support for smoking cessation in pregnancy: What are the barriers to stopping and which behavior change techniques can influence these? Application of theoretical domains framework. International Journal of Environmental Research and Public Health. 2018;**15**(2):piiE359. DOI: 10.3390/ijerph15020359

[50] Varghese S, Gasalberti D, Ahern K, Chang JC. An analysis of attitude toward infant sleep safety and SIDS risk reduction behavior among caregivers of newborns and infants. Journal of Perinatology. 2015;**35**(11):970-973

[51] Mitchell EA, Blair PS. SIDS prevention: 3000 lives saved but we can do better. The New Zealand Medical Journal. 2012;**125**(1359):50-57

[52] Jeffrey HE. Future directions in sudden unexpected death in infancy research. In: Duncan JR, Byard RW, editors. SIDS Sudden Infant and Early Childhood Death: The Past, the Present and the Future. Adelaide, Australia: University of Adelaide Press; 2018

[53] Dowling DA, Barsman SG, Forsythe P, Damato EG. Caring about Preemies' Safe Sleep (CaPSS): An educational program to improve adherence to safe sleep recommendations by mothers of preterm infants. The Journal of Perinatal & Neonatal Nursing. 2018;**32**(4):366-372

[54] Rubin R. Despite educational campaigns, US infants are still dying due to unsafe sleep conditions. JAMA. 2018;**319**(24):2466-2468

[55] Carlin RF, Abrams A, Mathews A, et al. The impact of health messages on maternal decisions about infant sleep position: A randomized controlled trial. Journal of Community Health. 2018;**43**:977-985. DOI: 10.1007/s10900-018-0514-0

[56] Wall SN, Lee AC, Niermeyer S, English M, Keenan WJ, Carlo W, et al.

Neonatal resuscitation in low-resource settings: What, who, and how to overcome challenges to scale up? International Journal of Gynaecology and Obstetrics. 2009;**107**(Supp. 1): S47-S64

[57] McGovern MC, Smith MBH. Causes of apparent life threatening events in infants: A systematic review. Archives of Disease in Childhood. 2004;**89**: 1043-1048

[58] Nehme Z, Namachivayam S, Forrest A, Butt W, Bernard S, Smith K. Trends in the incidence and outcome of paediatric out-of-hospital cardiac arrest: A 17-year observational study. Resuscitation. 2018 Jul;**128**:43-50. DOI: 10.1016/j.resuscitation.2018.04.030. Epub 2018 Ap. 25

[59] Goto Y, Maeda T, Goto Y. Impact of dispatcher-assisted bystander cardiopulmonary resuscitation on neurological outcomes in children with out-of-hospital cardiac arrests: A prospective, nationwide, population-based cohort study. Journal of the American Heart Association. 2014;**3**(3): e000499. DOI: 10.1161/JAHA.113. 000499

[60] Callahan JM, Fuchs SM, Committee on Paediatric Emergency Medicine. Advocating for life support training of children, parents, caregivers, school personnel, and the public. Pediatrics 2018;**141**(6). pii: e20180704. DOI: 10.1542/peds.2018-0704

[61] Chan GJ, Valsangkar B, Kajeepeta S, Boundy EO, Wall S. What is kangaroo mother care? Systematic review of the literature. Journal of Global Health. 2016;**6**(1):010701. DOI: 10.7189/ jogh.06.010701

[62] Boundy EO, Dastjerdi R, Spiegelman D, et al. Kangaroo mother care and neonatal outcomes: A meta-analysis. Pediatrics. 2016;**137**(1): e20152238. DOI: 10.1542/peds.2015-2238

[63] Sheridan E, Wright J, Small N, et al. Risk factors for congenital anomaly in a multiethnic birth cohort: An analysis of the Born in Bradford study. Lancet. 2013;**382**(9901):1350-1359. DOI: 10.1016/S0140-6736(13)61132-0. Epub 2013 Jul 4

[64] Kapurubandara S, Melov S, Shalou E, Alahakoon I. Consanguinity and associated perinatal outcomes, including stillbirth. The Australian & New Zealand Journal of Obstetrics & Gynaecology. 2016;**56**(6):599-604. DOI: 10.1111/ajo.12493. Epub 2016 Jul 11

[65] Institute of Medicine (US) Committee on Improving Birth Outcomes, Bale JR, Stoll BJ, Lucas AO, editors. Reducing Birth Defects: Meeting the Challenge in the Developing World. Washington (DC): National Academies Press (US); 2003. 3. Interventions to Reduce the Impact of Birth Defects. Available from: https://www.ncbi.nlm. nih.gov/books/NBK222083/

[66] Up to date—Preterm Birth: Risk Factors, Interventions for Risk Reduction and Maternal Prognosis. Available from: https://www.uptodate. com/contents/preterm-birth-risk-fac tors-interventions-for-risk-reduction-a nd-maternal-prognosis [Accessed: 15-10-2018]

[67] World Health Organization: Preterm Births. Available from: http:// www.who.int/news-room/fact-sheets/ detail/preterm-birth [Accessed 15-10-2018]

[68] Newnham JP, Dickinson JE, Hart RJ, Pennell CE, Arresse CA, Keelan JA. Strategies to prevent preterm birth. Frontiers in Immunology. 2014;**5**:584

[69] Baqui AH, Williams EK, Rosecrans AM, Agrawal PK, Ahmed S, Darmstadt GL, et al. Impact of an integrated nutrition and health programme on neonatal mortality in rural northern India. Bulletin of the World Health Organization. 2008;**86**:796-804

[70] Bhutta ZA, Memon ZA, Sooi S, Salat MS, Cousens S, Martines J. Implementing community-based perinatal care: Results from a pilot study in rural Pakistan. Bulletin of the World Health Organization. 2008;**86**:452-459

[71] Kumar V, Mohanty S, Kumar A, et al. Effect of community based behaviour change management on neonatal mortality in Shivgarh, Uttar Pradesh, India: A cluster randomised controlled trial. Lancet. 2008;**372**(9644):1151-1162

[72] Shealy KR, Li R, Benton-Davis S, Grummer-Strawn LM. The CDC Guide to Breastfeeding Interventions. Atlanta: U.S. Department of Health and Human Services, Centers for Disease Control and Prevention; 2005. Available from: https://www.cdc.gov/breastfeeding/pdf/breastfeeding_interventions.pdf

Printed in the USA
CPSIA information can be obtained
at www.ICGtesting.com
LVHW082132031024
792888LV00006B/29